MOONLIGHT
GRATITUDE

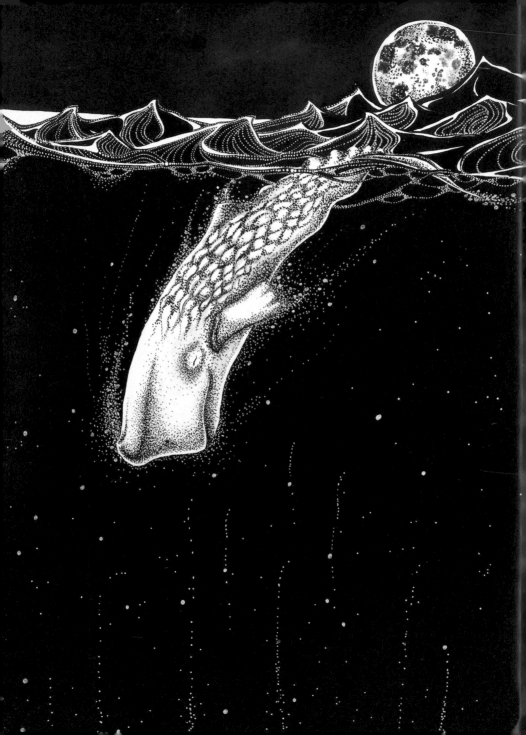

MOONLIGHT GRATITUDE

365 NIGHTTIME MEDITATIONS
FOR DFEP, TRANQUIL SLEEP
ALL YEAR LONG

EMILY SILVA

ROCK
POINT

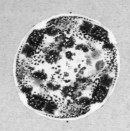

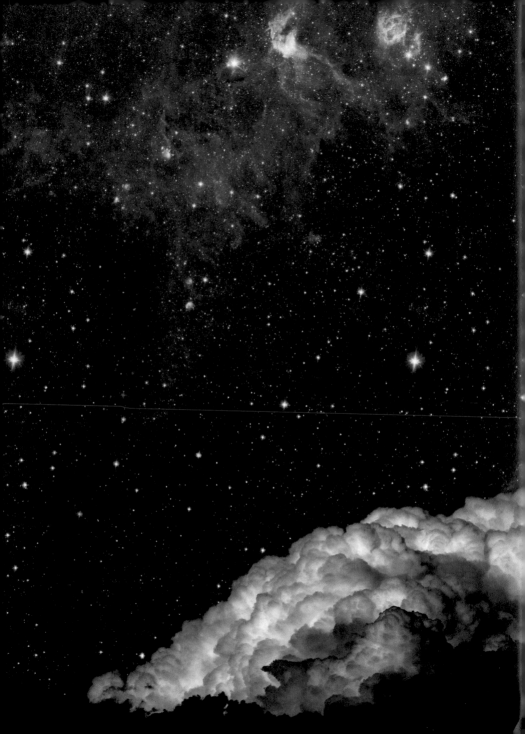

Introduction

I'm standing at a trailhead in Sedona looking at the moon. To my back, the sun is setting after a day full of thunder and lightning. I have a lump in my throat and tears in my eyes. A dream I have held in my heart for twenty-five years has come true. I have written a book: the one you're holding.

It amazes me how this process transpired. Someone found me to write a book of moonlight meditations. It couldn't be more perfect. Four years ago, I started setting intentions and practicing gratitude under a big full moon in Bali. It changed my life. I learned to trust the universe with my intentions and be immensely grateful for however they turned out.

My goal with this book is for the reader to find peace in these passages before falling asleep—to offer gratitude every night. The universe is abundant and full of goodness. Create a moment each day to say thank-you for the blessings that flow through to each one of us.

This evening, I am grateful to be in a dreamy place where I could complete this book and look up at the sky at a near full moon, offering my appreciation for this gift.

May your sleep be sound and may peace transcend your worry.

—EMILY SILVA

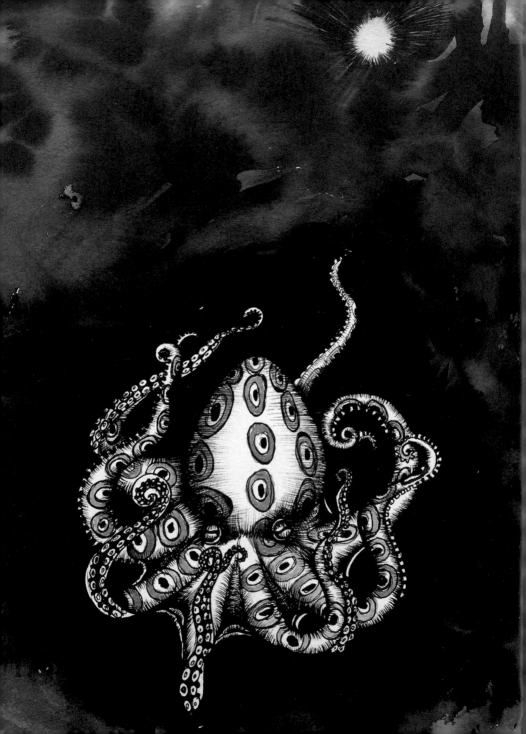

January 1

ILLUMINATION COMES FROM WITHIN and reflects outward. Sleep offers the time to recharge your inner light. As you drift off to sleep, reflect on how your light shone today and how others shared their lights with you. Breathe in this light and allow the day's shared illuminations to wash over you and cover you from the inside out. Offer gratitude and fall asleep knowing that this light is always glowing as you recharge your sparkle.

January 2

TODAY IS DONE; tomorrow has yet to arrive. This moment is all that matters. Be present and reflect on the good things that transpired today. Let go of the things that no longer serve you. This is the time to release and renew. Sleep restores. Focus on one thing that made you happy today and breathe in that memory. As you exhale, let everything else fall away. It is no longer needed.

———

January 3

AS THE MOON CASTS its silvery glow across the water, the ocean moves and responds to its pull. Tides rise and fall with the cycles of the moon. Be like the ocean, fluid and forgiving. Wash away whatever is holding you back. Forgive others and let go of the pain. Release all bitterness. Allow your breath to become rhythmic, like the waves on the shore, as you drift into a peaceful slumber. Breathe in forgiveness; breathe out bitterness.

January 4

EVEN WHEN THE NEW MOON is dark, the stars still shine. There is always light. Regardless of what you're going through, look for the light. When the light seems dim, find ways to fuel it. Think positive thoughts and offer gratitude. Allow the air and space to breathe so that the light can grow. What we nurture grows. Nurture your inner light, no matter how bright or dim. Remember that the stars still shine on the darkest nights. Whatever you're going through, you can still choose to shine.

January 5

A LIGHTHOUSE PROVIDES a guiding light for ships at sea. Its light shines in darkness, through fog, and during storms. Your inner light is your beacon through the dark times in life. To access your light, close your eyes, sit quietly, and listen to your breathing. Allow all thoughts to fade away. In stillness, your light can illuminate the truths that noise sometimes overwhelms. Like a ship coming safely to harbor, your soul will find peace in the darkness.

January 6

DEEP AND DARK, UNDER THE SEA, the moon's light reaches the depths and illuminates. The ocean is calm beneath the waves and life moves forward in natural rhythms. Underneath the stress and busyness of the day is your calm and natural rhythm. To access it, close your eyes and see a deep blue light covering you from your head all the way down to your toes. Release any tension and breathe into the release. Take time with this exercise. The goal is complete relaxation and access to your inner calm.

———

January 7

QUIETLY IN THE NIGHT, a sea turtle crawls onto the beach to lay her eggs in the sand. She finds a safe place for hatching and covers the eggs before heading back to sea, where she lets go of the outcome. Sleep is a time for dreams to propagate. The seed of a dream is the beginning of creation. When our minds rest, our subconscious has room to create, manifest, and deliver. Let go of the outcome and allow yourself to rest.

January 8

HAVE VAST, PROFOUND FAITH in manifesting your desires. Allow your dreams to take place; trust the universe with them. As you fall asleep, set an intention, release it to the universe, and be patient. Forces beyond your control are taking care of you and working to help you manifest your desires. Surrender and let go. Breathe in peace; breathe out control.

——————

January 9

HUSH NOW. As quiet envelops the night, it's time for slumber and dreams. In silence, our inner wisdom finds its voice. Connect with this silence and let go of your thoughts. You don't need them right now. In the void, dreams can take place. In the silence, ideas take shape. Quiet your mind by breathing in the silence and breathing out the noise. Listen to your breath as it goes in and out. Allow the breath to cover you in peace and quiet.

January 10

AFTER A LONG DAY IN THE SUN, the desert begins to cool. Sunset paints the sky with soft colors, becoming darker and darker until the stars showcase their brightness. In the absence of light, it is apparent how vast the universe is. Stars shoot across the heavens, leaving stardust behind them, continuing to shine up until the moment they leave the sky. We can emulate stars and decide to give off brilliance throughout life.

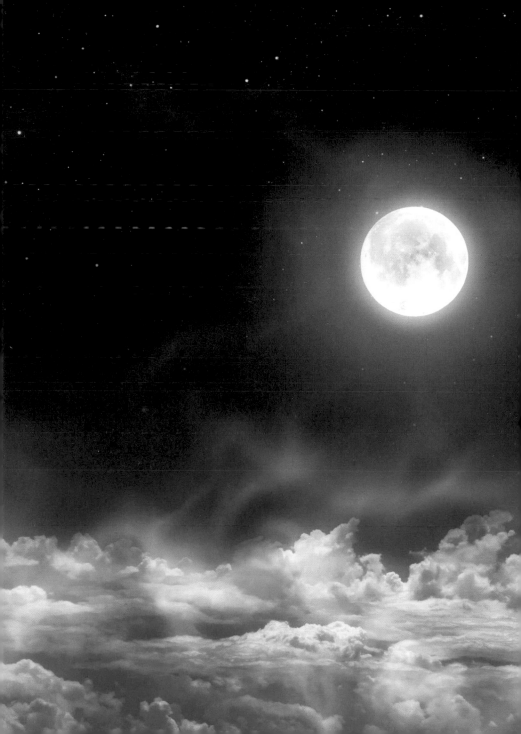

January 11

WHEN WINTER SETTLES IN, animals hibernate, away from the cold. The nights are longer and a chill sets in. Cover yourself with blankets and burrow in, like a rabbit in its hole. You are warm and protected from the cold. Send out gratitude for your bed, your home, and your safety. Underneath the covers, feel yourself drifting into a state of contented slumber.

———

January 12

RESPONDING TO PROBLEMS can cause a reactionary emotion. When we focus on the negative, this can mask the hope that dreams hold. If we choose to let problems flow in and out and we let go of outcomes, dreams have room to develop. Dreams can have power over problems by shifting the focus. Decide where you want to focus and redirect your thoughts.

January 13

JANUARY'S WOLF MOON: A wolf howls at the moon, paws embedded in the snow. A hunger gnaws within. Breath is visible as the howl fills the sky. This is the time to use instinct and intuition to go after what you want. When everything is covered with snow and is frozen, instincts become stronger and honed. A hunger can create urgency within the soul to hunt and seek. What are you yearning for? Allow your intuition to play a part in capturing that which you desire.

January 14

THE LOTUS DESCENDS under water when the day is done. Its bloom closes and rests. The next day, the lotus emerges and reopens refreshed, just as beautiful. Allow yourself to lie down on your bed and under your covers like a lotus. Let sleep take over and renewal to take place. When this happens you can awaken more vibrant and completely present for the day ahead. Emerge in the morning content with the rest that occurred.

January 15

THE CRESCENT MOON IS the moon of regeneration. It is the time of the month when the moon reflects the sun's light once more. Following a period of darkness, light reenters at a slow pace. Regeneration is a process. Notice where the light is beginning to shine. Don't force illumination. With time, we all fully shine once more. As a crescent moon shows us, everything does not need to be seen to be whole. Rest knowing that the light is regenerating in perfect time.

January 16

THE NIGHT IS QUIET. Welcome peace as darkness envelops what was once light. In this quiet, allow yourself to reflect. Whether routine or spontaneity shaped your day, this quiet space is the perfect place to reflect. What three things are you most grateful for today? Offer gratitude for each one of them. Think of the people you love and offer gratitude for them. End each day with a heart full of gratitude.

January 17

YOU CAN MAKE A WISH on a shooting star while standing on the ground and looking up. This image presents a dichotomy between what is ethereal and what is grounded. The ability to release a heart's desire to the universe while staying grounded is powerful. Balance the contrasts by staying grounded and remember what is important as your wishes and dreams actualize.

———

January 18

THE CRATERS ON THE MOON are places of damage, where asteroids hit the moon's surface. These supposed scars create depth and complexity, making the moon even more beautiful. No matter how many scars the moon has, it still reflects the sun's light, illuminating others. Our damage also creates depth and complexity in our souls. The key is to transform the pain into something beautiful. Don't hold on to the scar; let it heal and then appreciate the complexity it provides.

January 19

The fishermen know that the sea is dangerous and
the storm fearsome, but could never see that the dangers
were a reason to continue strolling on the beach.

—VINCENT VAN GOGH

THE MOST REWARDING THINGS in life have an element of risk. The greater the risk, the greater the reward. Vulnerability opens us up to the possibility of failure, but also greatness. Don't stand on the shore waiting for the fish; get on a boat, go out to sea, and go after what you really want.

January 20

IT WAS DARK AND QUIET. Two sisters lay side by side. One offered gratitude for the day. The other had a mind full of worry. One fell asleep and dreamt of peaceful things. The other remained awake, ruminating on the day's troubles. The next morning, one awoke refreshed and calm. The other awoke tired and anxious. At the end of the day, always count your blessings. This simple act does wonders in slumber and while awake.

———

January 21

There are years that ask questions and years that answer.
—ZORA NEALE HURSTON

EACH YEAR ARRIVES with questions and some years pass waiting for the answers to come. But the answers always come. Sometimes they do not arrive when we would like them to and all we can do is wait. If you are in a year of questions, allow the time to pass without force. Ease into the questions and embrace the answers when they arrive.

January 22

LIGHTS BEGIN TO ILLUMINATE the city as the sun sets. Only the brightest stars can be seen among the sparkle of the city. But all the stars are still shining. It is easy to allow our light to dim when we sense the brightness of others. But we have the power to shine as bright as possible so that our lights can be seen. Imagine how illuminated the planet would be if we all shone as bright as we could.

———

January 23

LONG INTO THE NIGHT, slumber grows deeper. Stillness occurs in the absence of the noise and haste of the day. Inside this silent rest, rejuvenation and dreams take place. Before you fall asleep, visualize a dream you would like to have come true. See yourself as if that dream is already happening. Spend a moment recognizing how it feels to be where you would like to be. Then offer gratitude as if it has already happened.

January 24

SELF-CARE IS IMPORTANT to be able to care for others. We can't extend to others what we can't extend to ourselves. Things like love, forgiveness, and compassion must be things we give ourselves. If you are longing for something from someone else, check to see whether you are extending it to yourself and nurture that need.

———

January 25

THE TIDES RESPOND to the gravitational pull of the moon. As the moon experiences its phases, changes occur miles away on Earth. All living things feel the power of its pull. Each month, we undergo changes. Some coincide with the moon's light. Take notice of what changes are happening right now. Rest knowing that it is natural and cyclical. Go with the flow. Don't resist the natural tugs that occur. Nothing is permanent. Honor your natural rhythms.

January 26

DEEP IN THE SEA, humpback whales sing their songs.
Sound travels far into the ocean's depths, carrying signals
to navigate, communicate, and attract mates. People record
and share these peaceful songs. The massive creature's
communication has a soothing effect. Our dreams can reveal
communications that lie deep within us, like the depths of
the sea. In slumber, our subconscious communicates with
us. Be open to receive what it has to say.

January 27

*Often when you think you're at the end of something,
you're at the beginning of something else.*
—FRED ROGERS

SOME THINGS END in the most unexpected ways. It
can be shocking and frustrating. Sorrow may follow. But if
things did not end, new things would not have the space
to enter. Remember a time when there was an ending
in life. Notice what took its place. Another beginning is
always waiting to happen.

January 28

A WAXING MOON REPRESENTS renewal after the darkness of the new moon. A crescent full of light grows from a place that was dark. As the light begins to grow and illuminate, the craters of the moon become more visible. Take time to reflect on what is being illuminated in your life right now. As the moon attains more light, consider what you would like to accomplish. Allow this time of restoration and growth to help you achieve a new goal.

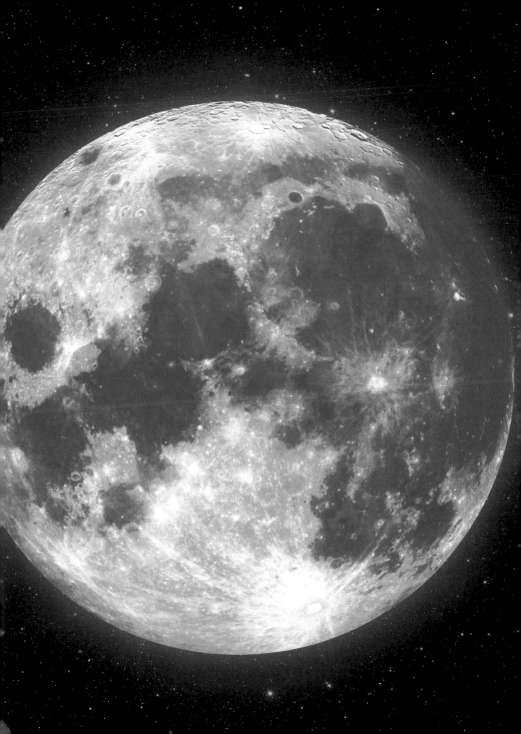

January 29

WORRY AND FEAR IMPRISON the mind. We can become slaves to the false truths they provide. When we act out of fear, we are not being true to ourselves. Write down your fears and notice where your anxiety is creating an inaccurate picture of reality. Identify the truth and embrace it with peace.

———

January 30

AS THE LIGHT from the moon disappears, the fullness of illumination begins to wane. Contemplate what was revealed under the radiance of the full moon. Surrender to the messages that were presented under the moon's light and let go of whatever is holding you back. Welcome this quiet time of waning light and consider the growth that is occurring. Receive the lessons and choose to expand as the light contracts.

January 31

We are tied to the ocean. And when we go back to the sea . . .
we are going back from whence we came.

—JOHN F. KENNEDY

THE OCEAN IS THE WOMB of the earth. All living things
are connected to it. Water is necessary for life from
birth to death. The tides move in rhythm with the cycles
of the moon that move with the cycles of the Earth.
Everything is cyclical and we are all connected. From
this understanding, extend love.

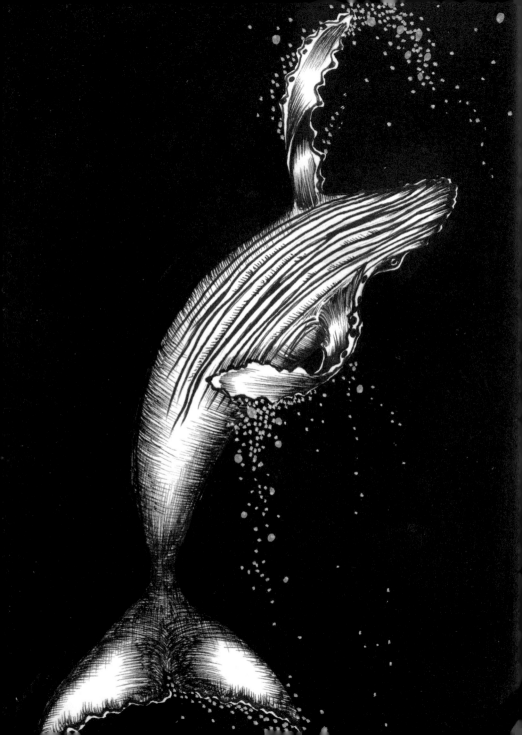

February 1

MOONLIGHT CASTS SHADOWS between the rows of trees in an orchard. Late at night it is quiet and peaceful here. The chirps of crickets interrupt the silence and the stars shine bright above. The shadows follow the moon as night progresses. There is nothing to do except be still. The stillness creates renewal for another day in the sun and for bearing fruit. But for now, in this moment, quiet is all that matters. Tonight, rest is all that matters.

February 2

A PART OF THE EARTH IS always illuminated. A sunset is a sunrise somewhere else. Everything is not necessarily dark. Even in our darkest moments, there is another side that is light. Looking at the bright side can be a lifeline when all seems dark. Even the moon and stars illuminate a night sky. There is always light. Search within for illumination. Imagine this light beginning to grow, shining hope into the darkness.

———

February 3

A FEELING OF DISCONTENT can cast a shadow in the soul. Longing for something that we don't have fixes our minds elsewhere. In this state, the shadows can permeate and settle. To counteract this mind-set, practice gratitude. On the hardest days, it is important to find things to be grateful for. Before falling asleep, think of three things you are grateful for today. Continue to think about these things. Allow your final thought of the night to be gratitude.

February 4

A DANCE IS a beautifully choreographed performance of moves and steps. Each element can create beautiful chaos without guidance. And each element is just as important as the others. Within the chaos, growth and wisdom occur. With practice, mastery is attained. We are all dancing stars in the choreography of the universe.

———

February 5

DURING THE RUSH OF THE DAY, it is easy to ignore the soul's calling. Routines take over, and it isn't until we settle into bed that we have time to hear what our souls have to say. Be grateful for the quiet moments at the end of the day and the busy moments too. Whether we spent our time at a job, helping others, or rushing around getting things done, these moments are creating something.

February 6

ANXIETY RESIDES IN anticipation and expectation of the unknown. There will always be an unknown. It is important to anchor in the present moment. Breathe into what is happening at this very moment. Let go of the need to know. Answers will be revealed in due time.

February 7

THE EVERGREEN PERPETUALLY displays its color whatever the season. It is constant, strong, and fragrant. Its best self is not deterred by environmental factors; it continues to grow. Even in the harshest winter cold, the evergreen relies on its inner resources to survive. When you are going through a difficult season, look inside and identify your inner resources. Lean into the strength they provide. Breathe in this strength; breathe out self-defeat.

———

February 8

WE CANNOT CONTROL what happens. When we embrace the present moment and infuse it with love and positive energy, we raise the vibration of the planet. If each person infused the present moment with love and positivity, imagine the shift that would occur. Create an inner shift by offering love and gratitude to yourself and all you encountered today.

February 9

UNCONDITIONAL LOVE IS available to us at all times.
The universe shows us love through the blooming of a
flower, a beautiful sunset, and kind words from a friend.
Even on the hardest days, there is love. When our needs
are met, there is love. When someone offers help, there is
love. As you drift off to sleep, think about all the ways you
notice love in your life. Feel your heart radiate this love.

———

February 10

SWOOPING HIGH ABOVE THE TREES, an owl sees
clearly in the dark. By using its powerful eyesight and
hearing, an owl can be secretive in its approach to prey.
Because owls can see what others may not, they are often
symbols for wisdom and insight. Without the distractions
of the day, night allows us the time to contemplate what
we may have missed. After a few moments in stillness,
recognize what insights are revealed. Soar above any
problems with your newfound wisdom.

February 11

OUT IN THE MIDDLE of the ocean, a sailor looks west as the sun sets low beyond the horizon. Pink sunsets indicate fair weather for the day to come. After a long day at sea, the pink sky is comforting. Not every day is going to be difficult. Allow the stress of the day to melt away. Imagine a pink sunset as you drift toward sleep. Look forward to the promise of a beautiful day to come.

———

February 12

Find a place inside where there's joy,
and the joy will burn out the pain.
—JOSEPH CAMPBELL

THE SUN BURNS OFF the fog after it has had time to hang low and cover the earth with its opaque veil. There is always sunlight behind the thickest fog. When sorrows enshroud us, we can have hope knowing joy is always on the other side. Through the pain and suffering, joy is trying to make its way back to your soul.

February 13

FEBRUARY'S SNOW MOON: The moon illuminates the snow-covered earth. Everything is insulated by winter's snowfall. A hush is heard as the snowflakes reach the ground. The cold air seems to heighten the moonlight's reflection on the white ground. Silver light shines on a vast white canvas. Underneath, everything is frozen and fallow. Now is the time to rest and recover. Soon, spring will arrive and growth will accelerate. But for now, allow yourself to rest.

February 14

PATIENCE IS A RESULT of waiting. But waiting can be hard to endure. The universe provides lessons in patience to challenge our endurance. Strength is a product of perseverance. Try to exhibit patience in the process. Being present and focusing on the current moment helps alleviate the longing for the future. When you catch yourself feeling a familiar twinge of impatience, breathe into the present moment and focus on one thing that makes today lovely.

February 15

Finish each day before you begin the next, and
interpose a solid wall of sleep between two.

—RALPH WALDO EMERSON

EVENING IS THE TIME to wind down from the day.
Tomorrow does not need your attention until you awaken.
Finish your day with gratitude and peace. If there is
anything left undone, finish it or leave it for another day.
Create the space for sleep to occur. Tomorrow will come
in its own time.

February 16

A DIAMOND HOLDS great value after years under intense pressure. For the diamond to be revealed, hard work must take place. The process can take a long time and may seem tedious. Sometimes we have to undergo increased pressure—and our actions, not reactions, reveal the worth we have inside. If we merely reacted to pressure, we would give up long before the treasure is revealed. Trials reveal our inner strength and beauty, and in the end, you will shine like a diamond.

———

February 17

TAKE A MOMENT TO REFLECT on the people in your life who brought happiness into your day. Offer gratitude for each one of them. Notice how they created expansion in your heart and send them love as you offer gratitude. Every day, notice who brought joy—and resolve to do the same for others.

February 18

Beauty appears when one feels deeply,
and art is an act of total attention.
—DOROTHEA LANGE

WHEN WE COME ACROSS a thing of beauty, a state of awe often takes place. Giving beauty our complete attention can deepen the connection to that moment. An open mind, ready to see and feel, will notice such instances more easily. To find beauty, open your mind and soul to feeling deeply. Connect with the reverence and awe that is available every day.

February 19

SLOWLY, A COYOTE MAKES its way across the desert, guided by moonlight. In Navajo legend, he is credited for the formation of the Milky Way due to his impatience with waiting for the constellations to take shape. He looks up at the stars and howls as the moon, forlorn that his impatience did not create a celestial coyote. Like the coyote, we need to be careful when we are creating. Impatience breeds unfinished work. Be patient with your creations. In time, magnificence will be revealed.

February 20

If you care about what you do and work hard at it,
there isn't anything you can't do if you want to.
—JIM HENSON

THE WORK WE DO can emulate our passions, integrity, and drive. All work deserves care, and if we focus enough, we can find work that we deeply care about. Hard work pays off when care is given. There is a blessing in having a job to complete. Be grateful for the work you did today and rest well to prepare for tomorrow.

———

February 21

SITTING UNDER A FULL MOON'S LIGHT is peaceful and empowering. Look up at the moon; notice how it uses the sun's light to illuminate and glow. Contemplate how you can reflect the moon's reflection of the sun to do the same. Breathe in radiance and breathe out darkness. Imagine yourself shining brightly, lighting up any dim or dark places that surround you. Pay attention to what your light reveals and resolve to continue to shed light in this space.

February 22

SPENDING TIME ALONE IS not necessarily loneliness. Solitude can be empowering. Loneliness can drain us because of longing and expectation. When alone, creating a state of presence can transform loneliness into the beauty of solitude. To create this state, focus on the present moment and where you are. Offer gratitude for this moment and anything else that is good and lovely. Continue to be present, not letting your mind ruminate on other times. All that matters is right here, right now.

February 23

A ruffled mind makes a restless pillow.
—CHARLOTTE BRONTË

SLEEP DOES NOT COME easily when our minds are restless and full of worry. Becoming still and grounded before slumber can help alleviate the busyness of the mind. Make sure to turn off and put away stimuli before you go to sleep. Keep the bedroom as a sanctuary where outside influences, like electronics, aren't invited. Take the time to still the mind through meditation; this will set the stage for quiet and rest.

February 24

THE MORE OUTER SPACE IS EXPLORED, the
more apparent it becomes that we have much to learn.
The universe is vast and our reality is a tiny dot. This
knowledge highlights the grandeur and greatness of
something much bigger and more powerful than we are.
Think about this force and about any issues that may
be flooding your mind. See that whatever you are going
through is an exchange of energy. Infuse any nervous
energy with calm, healing energy, knowing that the
universe has everything under control.

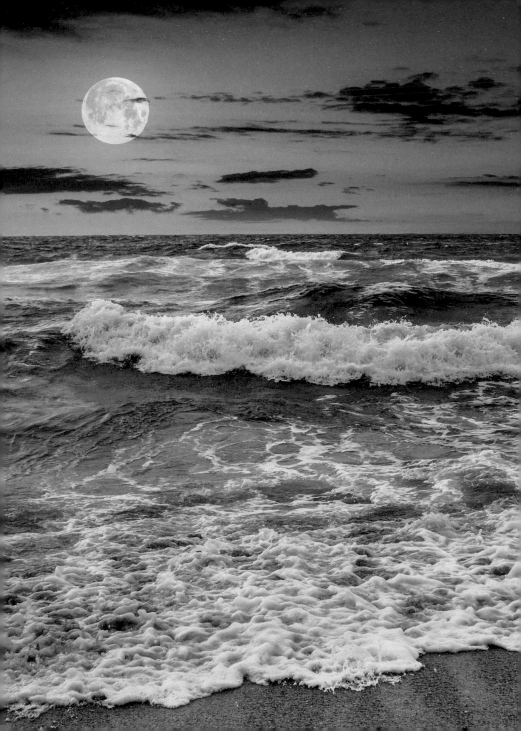

February 25

That is happiness; to be dissolved into something complete and
great. When it comes to one, it comes as naturally as sleep.

—WILLA CATHER

SURRENDERING TO OUR life's purpose brings
happiness and contentment. Be open to what life wants
from you. Look for where your soul lights up and ignites
purpose within. Every person has something they
are good at. Embrace your natural strengths and the
greatness that results.

———

February 26

LIGHTS FLASH, GUIDING PLANES as they depart
and arrive. Looking over an airport at night can be
mesmerizing, as the lights on the ground direct air traffic.
Whether we are leaving something behind or arriving at a
new understanding, a guiding light within us helps direct
our paths. Take time to center and connect with your
breath; this can bring you back on course and illuminate
your direction.

February 27

Let everything happen to you: beauty and terror.
Just keep going. No feeling is final.

—RAINER MARIA RILKE

EVERYTHING PASSES EVENTUALLY. There is no finality to life, as it keeps going on. Even after we pass on, we continue as dust and energy radiated. Allow things to come and go without attachment and expectation, for therein lies the pain. Release, let go, move on. Exhale.

February 28/29

THE UNKNOWN CAN CREATE a sense of feeling out of control of circumstances and outcomes. When we hold on to our controlling tendencies, anxiety sets in. It is important to ground ourselves in the present moment, and although the outcome is a mystery, to anticipate it with excitement instead of worry. The mystery itself is a beautiful thing. Be grateful for the process and notice the beauty in the unveiling of what is to come.

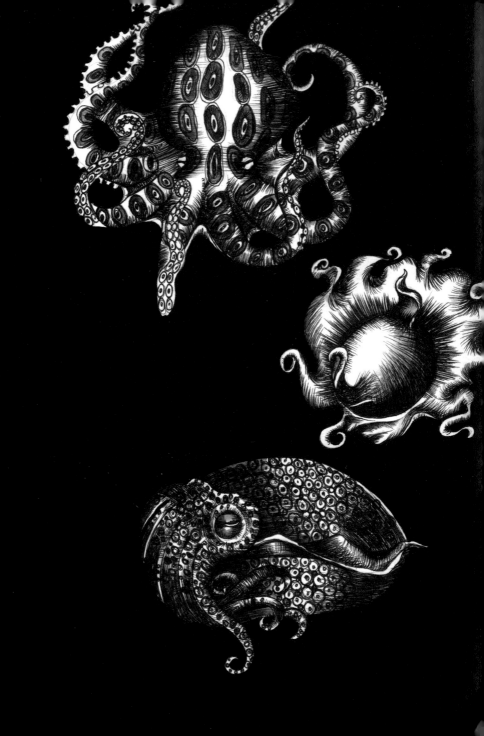

March 1

DEEP IN THE OCEAN, an octopus shape-shifts, changing with its environment. It is fluid like its ocean home and it adapts to new circumstances. As the moon changes the ocean's tide, the octopus adapts, waxing and waning in unison. Even though the moon is high above the ocean, an octopus is aware of the moon's pull and adjusts. This is a picture of being aware of our surroundings and of our higher self. Find the balance and harmony between these two needs. Give and take as needed.

March 2

SIMPLICITY CREATES A SENSE of order. When things feel as if they are out of control, it is easy to ignore the tiny things that keep life in order. Instead of overlooking tasks, find comfort in the ability to complete them. Simple tasks can be grounding during a chaotic time. Start by creating a sacred space in your bedroom. Put clothes away before you get into the bed you made when you woke up. Find order amid the chaos.

———

March 3

EVERY DAY WE HAVE a choice about how to use our time. We can fill our hours with things that uplift us or things that create atrophy. Take a few moments to reflect on how you spent your day. Our energy is a gauge that mirrors how we fill our time. Do you feel happy and energized or sad and depleted? Think about moments when your energy was positive and offer gratitude. Think of the moments when you felt depleted and let them go. Create the space for positive energy to flow.

March 4

THERE IS A PLAN FOR your life. Nothing is a mistake. What comes next will be revealed in due time. Surrender to the unknown. It is not necessary to know everything at all times. Let go of any expectations and attachments to the outcome. The only thing that is important right now is this moment. Be present and breathe peace into the unknown. Exhale all stress and anxiety. Don't resist the process; trust the process.

March 5

The world breaks everyone, and afterward,
some are strong at the broken places.
—ERNEST HEMINGWAY

SOME HARDSHIPS ARE UNAVOIDABLE. Some people break under the pressure only to come out stronger and wiser. Others submit to the pain and a vortex of brokenness is created. When difficulties arise, there is often an opportunity to gain strength. Lean on others for support and ask for help. Let the break help create resilience and newfound courage.

March 6

THE NEW MOON CREATES a clean slate, a place where dreams and intentions have room to grow. This is the time to let go of all that is no longer serving us. Recognize what is holding back the growth that is waiting to emerge. When we recognize what is stifling growth, we can choose to regain power and let it go. Toss whatever it is to the wind and allow it to be carried away—far, far away. Release what is holding you back and appreciate the freedom in the release.

March 7

HIGH ABOVE THE CLOUDS, an airplane flies into the sunset. Warm colors fill the plane's cabin while the sun's final rays kiss the sky. As night descends, the moon and stars become more visible. Watching night fall in the sky is magical. Light slowly becomes dimmer, allowing heavenly bodies to shine. As the lights dim tonight, notice how you shine. Embrace the illumination that darkness reveals. Just like the night sky, your shine is always present.

March 8

CHILDREN PLAYING NEAR the ocean on top of a hill see fog rolling in from the water. The fog sets in above their game, creating a light drizzle. Instead of complaining, the children continue their game. Soon after, the fog rolls back to sea. Our emotions are like fog, rolling in and out. When we feel troubled, we can choose to continue to play and live with joy and astonishment. Our childlike wonder can help lift the fog in our lives.

————

March 9

RELAXED IN A DREAM STATE, the mind is able to explore. Without the boundaries of consciousness our soul speaks, leaving remnants when we awaken. Even during the day, dream states can explore the longings of the soul. When the soul speaks, listen. Our judgments and conditioning create limitations. To quiet the mind, practice breathing long, measured breaths, in and out. Quiet the mind and prepare for a night of limitless dreaming.

March 10

HIGH ON THE TOP OF A MOUNTAIN, snow slowly melts and trickles its way down. As it gains momentum and volume, a river forms and continues to flow all the way to the edge of a cliff, where it cascades down the mountainside. The waterfall continues its way to the sea. From frozen to flowing, the cycle continues. Endings are also beginnings, and by letting go and falling down, the cycle can continue. Falling can also be a beginning. Look for the beauty in each stage and in letting go.

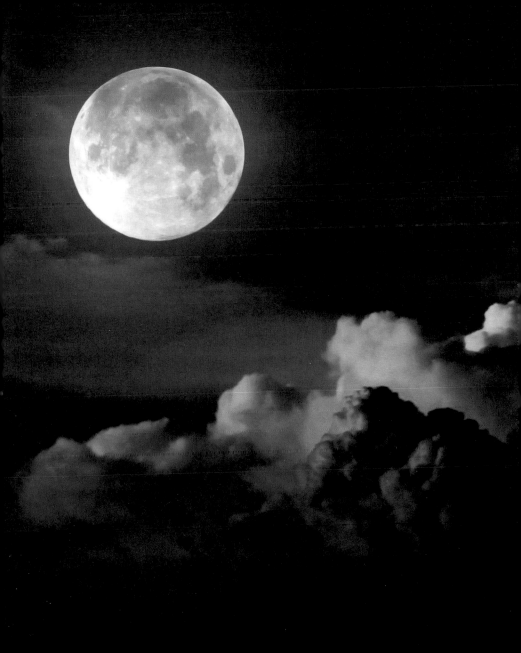

March 11

The sea, once it casts its spell, holds one in
its net of wonder forever.
—JACQUES COUSTEAU

TO BE IN THE PRESENCE of the sea is powerful. As
the waves crash, their power can be felt in the soul. In
the middle of the ocean, the vastness creates a sense of
awe. Underwater, the presence of vibrant life commands
wonder. After one encounter, it is difficult to forget or
deny the power of the sea.

March 12

FOG ROLLS IN AND VEILS the sun before the last
rays of the day. Through the veil, light can still be seen,
but it appears dimmer. Even though the fog creates a
visual barrier, the sun's rays are still powerful and light
infiltrates the cover. When we go through ambiguous
times, it can feel like we're in a fog. Although we would
prefer to have a clear picture, the answer is hidden. Allow
the light to shine on the situation. Just as fog eventually
rolls away, so will the answer be revealed.

March 13

MARCH'S WORM MOON: As the ground begins to thaw, making a fertile home for new seeds, worms begin to move the earth. The soil is being prepared for the sowing of seeds. What seeds are you planting in your life? Reflect on what you would like to plant spiritually. Think about what you would like to harvest in your life six months from now. Make an intention to plant those seeds and allow the space and time for growth.

March 14

THE MANIFESTATION OF something we desire is more joyful when it is realized. Setting intentions communicates our deepest desires to the universe. When the moon is full, we can notice what is becoming illuminated in our lives. Look back on the past few months and recognize any desires that have manifested. Acknowledge the work you completed to help this happen and notice how the universe played a part in delivering your intentions. Offer gratitude for both parts working together in the actualization of your dreams.

March 15

ONE OF THE GREATEST GIFTS we can give to each other is to listen. Sitting with someone and really taking the energy to listen with love and compassion is an art and a gift. Think of a time when you felt that someone truly listened to you. Remember how it felt to be truly heard. To extend this gift, we need to open our hearts and ears to hear the other person without interruption. Think of one person you can extend this gift to and visualize yourself creating a sacred place for this to happen.

March 16

LIKE A SOOTHING LULLABY, the rain falls onto the roof. As it beats down, it creates a rhythm. Each drop has its place in nature's orchestra. The tiniest raindrop makes a difference to nature's lullaby. If you are feeling small and insignificant, think about each raindrop. You are just as important to the rhythm of life. Without your contribution, the song would be missing a beat. You are not only a part of the song; your life is a song.

March 17

GONE TOO SOON ARE the ones we love. Into the ether their souls ascend as we stay here to feel the loss. The pang of loss resides in our hearts, in our bellies, even on our skin. Some days are easier than others, but the memories of our loved ones remain. Tonight, if a certain memory seems to linger, acknowledge its presence, notice where it affects you, and appreciate the person's presence in your life. Allow the memory to cultivate not sorrow, but gratitude.

March 18

A CACTUS GROWS FLOWERS as well as spines. One adorns, other protects. The flower symbolizes the ability to become beautiful in harsh conditions. The spines protect against predators, yet the flower still blooms. When we go through difficult situations, it is easy to put a protective wall around our hearts. But we can be more like the flower and continue to grow and showcase the beauty we have, despite hardships.

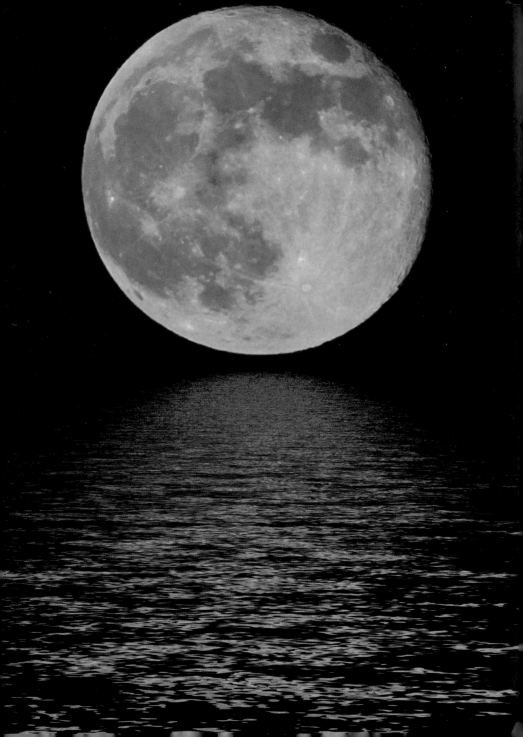

March 19

TO TRUST IS TO LET GO and know that everything is working out just the way it needs to be. This can be a scary concept, especially when the urge to control is strong. The key is to release your attachment to the outcome and have faith that all the work you have been doing will pay off. Sometimes the answers are not what we would like to hear, but they only bring us closer to where we need to be.

March 20

Have courage for the great sorrows of life and patience for the small ones; and when you have laboriously accomplished your daily tasks, go to sleep in peace. God is awake.

—VICTOR HUGO

SORROWS COME AND GO, and the growth they bring teaches us how strong we have become. Courage expands as we embrace the bravery that vulnerability requires. Patience develops while we wait for outcomes to transpire. Through all of the trials, a divine hand is helping us through each one.

———

March 21

HAPPINESS SPROUTS INTERNALLY when positive thoughts water the seeds of intention. Creating a life plan and visualizing it helps intentions take root. The more your focus is positive, the larger the sprout can grow. Take steps toward actualizing dreams to help solidify growth and direction. When you focus your attention, the universe collaborates to deliver the intention. Before you drift off to sleep, hold your vision in your mind and send it positive thoughts. Then, let it go and let the universe take over.

March 22

BELIEFS ARE STRONGER THAN WORRIES. While worries come and go, beliefs take root in our lives and flourish from the nutrition we give them over time. Sometimes, we convince ourselves that worries are beliefs, but when we examine them, they show how flimsy they are. As you go to sleep, take a moment to appreciate the lasting strength behind the things you truly believe.

———

March 23

ARE YOU WAITING for something to happen? Have you been waiting for an answer? Timing is everything. Just like the tide responds to the pull of the moon at the perfect time, allow the ebb and flow of life to happen. There will be times of plenty and of scarcity, but they will even out. When hardships occur, look for strength and rely on your resources to get through. Meditate, ask for help, and trust that your needs are being provided for.

March 24

EXCITEMENT CAN CLOAK ITSELF as fear, especially when it is paired with anxiety. In the process of waiting, we create stories in our minds about the outcome or process. This anticipatory excitement can become anxiety if we allow our minds to create worrisome tales. It is important to stay present and detach from the outcome. Instead of projecting into the future, anchor your thoughts in the here and now. The outcome will manifest when the time is right.

———

March 25

OUR THOUGHTS HAVE a lot of power and positive or negative thoughts affect our attitudes. Think about times when your thoughts were flooded with positivity. Do the same about times when your thoughts were mainly negative. The way to train our minds to stay positive is to catch the negative thoughts when they arise. Stop the thought and reframe it into something positive. Slowly, this process can change the way you think and even react.

March 26

Happiness is not a possession to be prized,
it is a quality of thought, a state of mind.

—DAPHNE DU MAURIER

TO BE HAPPY—REALLY HAPPY—we must choose to
be in that state of mind. Our thoughts generate our
moods and perspectives. When something happens,
we have the choice to see it as positive or negative. If
negative thoughts come up, notice the pattern, stop, and
reframe them positively. There is always a bright side.

March 27

A WAVE SWELLS before it breaks. Energy generated
offshore, miles away, causes the wave to rise. At
the moment of the swell, all that energy has been
accumulated into a powerful, beautiful force. When a
wave breaks, it releases miles and miles of energetic
buildup. A small drop in the ocean can create ripples and
then waves. Think about the energy you are emitting and
the type of waves you create.

March 28

The Soul should always stand ajar, That if the heaven inquire,
He will not be obliged to wait, Or shy of troubling her.

—EMILY DICKINSON

OPENNESS IS A PLACE to be filled. There is a
vulnerability in being open and ready to receive. When
things are closed down, nothing can enter; a place that is
open then becomes a void. The things that can fill this place
might be sad, but also wonderful and magnetic. Stay open
and trust that the universe wants to deliver awe.

———

March 29

IN AN ORCHESTRA, each instrument has its place and
sound. The conductor cues musicians at just the right
moment, when their instruments will make the most
impact. Musicians trust not only the conductor, but their
instincts as well. These instincts have been honed through
years of practice. Our instinct is a small voice inside that
guides us. The universe is like a conductor, helping us
notice where and when we can be most effective. Our
intuition is our gift from the universe. It is like an inner
compass, guiding and helping us.

March 30

THE MOST IMPORTANT MOMENT in your life is right now. Make the most of this moment. If you are getting ready to sleep, the state of rest is the most amazing state right now. Whatever you are doing, try to make it the best version of that activity. Practicing mindfulness and being present create a state of awe that allows us to revel in what is in front of us. Instead of focusing on what has passed or what is next, find wonder in your current moment and state.

———

March 31

SPRING IS THE TIME when the ground has thawed after the cold of winter. The soil is tilled and ready for the planting of seeds. Creating an environment conducive to growth is necessary for the seeds' success. As spring arrives, think about the seeds you would like to plant in your life and then create an environment for growth. If there is anything you need to let go in order for your seeds to thrive, now is the time to release and plant them.

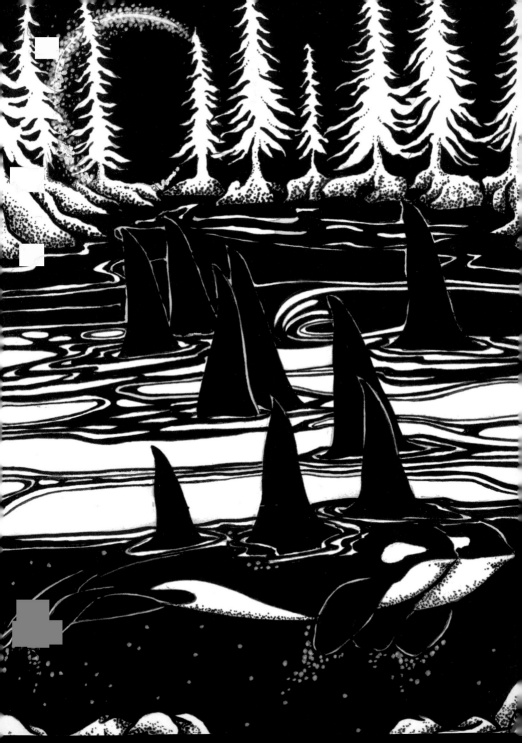

April 1

ON A CALM EVENING, a mist settles above the sea.
Slowly, something black appears, barely breaking the
calmness of the water. An orca surfaces, and then two
more rise up beside it. They glide gracefully side by side.
The sea remains calm in the presence of their power
and everything coexists peacefully. When great things
happen, they need not break our sense of tranquility.
Learning to allow things to happen and pass requires
mindfulness and acceptance. Find peace and harmony
when disruption looms.

April 2

IN THE SPRING, we take time to rid our closets and homes of clutter that accumulated during the winter. Spring cleaning creates the sense of a blank slate and starting anew. It is important to do the same for our minds and bodies. We can accumulate clutter spiritually and physically through emotions we have held on to, beliefs that no longer serve us and negative eating habits that need amending. Make a list of all that you would like to clear out of your mental, physical, and emotional space. Visualize the outcome. Breathe in the freedom and expansion.

April 3

I said to my soul, be still, and wait without hope,
For hope would be hope for the wrong thing.
—T. S. ELIOT

HOPE WITH EXPECTATIONS CAN lead to disappointment. Expectations create an invisible measurement of an unknown outcome. Waiting can be difficult, and finding a place of stillness can help ease the discomfort of anxiety. The soul finds balance in stillness. Hope can arise from this quiet place when we set aside expectations.

April 4

LIKE A WOMB, the sway of the ocean creates a safe cocoon where sea creatures can sleep. Waves pulse back and forth, up and down, rocking the ocean to sleep. Growth and transformation occur in cocoons and wombs. A body at rest does not stop changing. As you fall asleep tonight, allow your blankets to enfold you. Recognize the growth that will take place during your rest and give thanks.

April 5

EACH LIFE HAS A MOLD of its own and it is up to you to fashion yours the way you desire. Dreams and wishes are the substances that create outcomes. By visualizing what you want your life to look like, you generate energy and the universe responds.

April 6

WHEN WE ARE WOUNDED and heal, we have the opportunity to offer support and understanding to others who are going through similar situations. It is powerful to understand that your pain can create a healer within you. Wisdom has been passed down for ages. Without the experience of pain and suffering, wisdom would lack depth. Celebrate overcoming pain and create a space for healing within. From this place your inner light will illuminate.

April 7

THE MOON HAS FEMININE ENERGY. Its light is a soft reflection of the sun's own powerful light. The moon receives and gives back by illuminating what was dark. The cycles of the Earth are dependent on the moon, as a child is dependent on his or her mother. As the moon cycles, it cues the tides and even our bodies about when to rise, fall, and react. As the moon receives light, allow yourself to receive illumination too. Sit under the light of the moon and be open.

April 8

OVERNIGHT, A TREE CREATES blossoms that wait until morning to open. The blossoms are a work in progress, requiring time to form and bud. When it is time to reveal the blossoms' beauty, the tree stands tall, proud of its colorful display. This is only a step in bearing fruit, but each step is beautiful. Take a moment to embrace the stage you are at now. Remember that with time, the process will be complete.

April 9

It is a common experience that a problem difficult at night is resolved in the morning after the committee of sleep has worked on it.

—JOHN STEINBECK

SLEEP NOW; DON'T WORRY about what has happened or what is to come. You cannot solve problems at this moment. Let them go. Allow your mind to settle down by releasing the grasp on expectations and outcomes. What will be is already in the works. Breathe out the need to know and drift peacefully to sleep.

April 10

THE MOON WANTED TO LEARN TO DANCE, but being so large, it thought dancing was impossible. It rotated around the Earth and watched people dancing in its silver light. One day the moon looked down over the ocean and noticed its reflections swaying in the waves. Its unlikely partner, the ocean, complemented the moon's desire to dance. The waves moved according to the moon's pull. Not all partnerships are what we might have imagined. Keep your heart open with acceptance and gratitude.

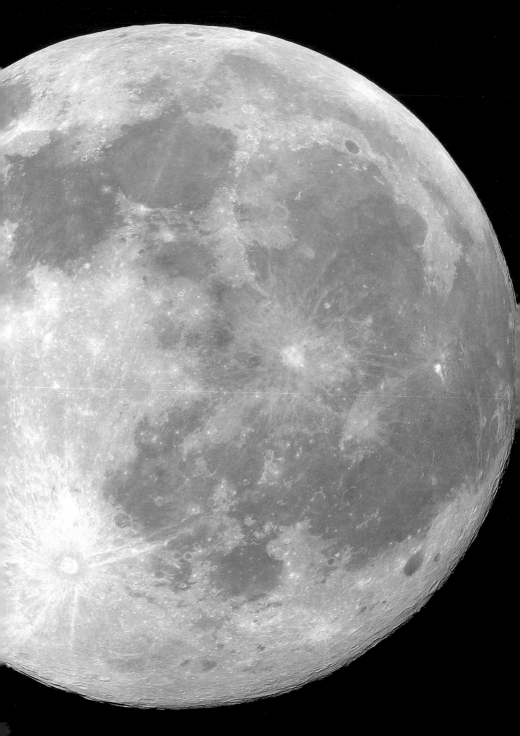

April 11

WHAT WE PAY ATTENTION TO GROWS. If our thoughts are positive, we notice more positivity. The same can be said about negative thoughts. If we focus on the negative, the positive may go unseen. Practicing gratitude can alleviate the tendency to focus on the unpleasant things in life. Create a habit of saying thank-you as often as possible. Little gifts are all around. Cultivate positivity with appreciation and it will flourish.

———

April 12

There are things known and there are things unknown, and in between are the doors of perception.

—ALDOUS HUXLEY

WHAT WE KNOW TO BE TRUE was once only a perception. As facts and opinions surface, we have the ability to choose how we want to see each thing. If there is a great unknown right now, choose the perspective that will serve the situation best. All things will be revealed in due time.

April 13

APRIL'S PLANTER'S MOON: Now that the ground has thawed, the first blooms of spring are blossoming on trees and on the ground. Take note of what is sprouting in your life. Soon the seeds you planted will come to fruition. This is the time to make sure that no weeds are growing where you intended seeds to take root. Let go of what impedes growth. Water your intentions with gratitude and purpose. Be open to receive the rain of blessings that will fall.

April 14

DREAMS CAN BE ATTAINED if we believe. Once there were no footprints on the moon or flags on top of Mount Everest. Someone dreamed of these feats and actualized their dreams with hard work and determination. Whatever your dream is, it too can happen. Visualize yourself as if the dream has already come true. Drift off to sleep with this vision in your mind's eye.

April 15

ALONG A TRAIL, under the moonlight, two hikers ascend a mountain. The night air cools their skin. The moonlight casts shadows along the trail and highlights each tree and rock along the path. It is quiet and peaceful with only the sound of the hikers' steps. There is no rush as the moon steadily illuminates the climb. At the top, the moon seems closer and the only shadows belong to the two companions. They look up to the moon in quiet appreciation.

April 16

CREATIVITY RESIDES in each and every one of us. It takes shape in countless forms and manifests itself in many ways, including through word, song, invention, and artwork. Creators must let go of control to allow their muse to visit and inspire. Creativity thrives in release and contracts with control. To find your creative flow, release your grasp on the outcome. Trust the process and allow inspiration to have its way. Remove restrictions and feel free.

April 17

DOUBT CAN STEAL OUR FOCUS on the divine. Where there is fear and hesitation, there is little room for trust or divine guidance. Interrupt this pattern with prayer and meditation. If something makes you feel uneasy and you desire peace, ask for divine guidance. Seek the answers within. Doubt is fear talking, but faith can speak louder if we listen. In stillness the answers will be revealed. Breathe in peace and stillness, breathe out doubt and fear. Miracles happen when people believe they are possible.

April 18

BRIGHT SHOCKS OF LIGHT intermittently strike across the night sky over the plains. Lightning creates powerful streaks, illuminating a dark sky. Each bolt has strength and ferocity. The lightning commands attention and inspires awe; even the clouds rumble with thunder in response. Sometimes when we find ourselves in a dark place, enlightenment comes sporadically. Pay attention and take action when needed. The storm will pass and the big picture will become clear.

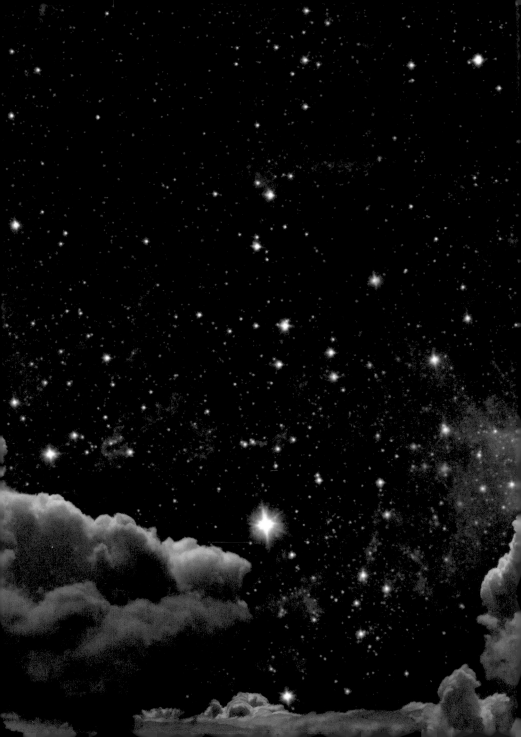

April 19

Difficult times have helped me to understand better than
before, how infinitely rich and beautiful life is in every way,
and that so many things that one goes worrying about are
of no importance whatsoever.

—ISAK DINESEN

WORRY EATS UP PRECIOUS TIME from the things that
actually matter. Behind the anxiety are beautiful things
waiting to be discovered. Find relief from everyday
troubles by taking time to be in the present moment.
Look for the beauty of that instant.

April 20

AS THE MOON ILLUMINATES the darkness of night, it unveils shadows. Our souls also have shadows that can become visible in the dark. Frustrations that have festered and grown can use this light. If you face something painful or frustrating, allow light to shine. Look at it from another perspective. Approach the person who hurt or frustrated you with love. Offer understanding and forgiveness. Through this, peace can be restored and resentment can dissipate.

———

April 21

THERE IS NO LONGER NEED to worry about the day that is ending. What is done is done. Right now I have the power to reset and remove all negative thoughts and feelings before I sleep. As I breathe in, I allow peace and tranquility to flood my being. As I exhale, I release all tension and angst; it no longer serves me. I am calm. I invite harmony and balance back in.

April 22

THE MOON'S ENERGY HAS a magnetic pull on the soul.
Its cycles create an ebb and flow in water as well as in
our bodies. As the moon becomes full, we can feel a
tug within. Like a wolf that howls in the moonlight, our
innermost longings make themselves known. It is almost
impossible to ignore the moon's magnetism. What are
you feeling pulled toward and pulled away from? What are
you attracting in your life? If there is any imbalance, let go
of what is weighing you down and become a magnet for
what your soul truly desires.

April 23

Silence is the sleep that nourishes wisdom.
—FRANCIS BACON

NOISE STIMULATES AND AWAKENS the senses. Slumber
requires silence and calm. It is important to silence the body
and mind before going to bed. Create the time to quiet the
mind and breathe in and out. Let the breath calm your body
from head to toe. Scan your body and notice any places that
need extra calming breaths; send stillness to them.

April 24

OFFERING GRACE IS AN EXTENSION of acceptance from one heart to another. By accepting and loving each and every creature, the universe is the ultimate example of grace. There is grace in forgiveness and letting go. Think of a hand gripping onto something. The posture is powerful and rigid. But if the hand releases its grasp and lets each finger fall naturally, the movement is more graceful and natural. Let go of your grasp, offering grace to yourself and to others.

April 25

FREEDOM FEELS AS LIGHT as a feather that floats carelessly with the breeze. As the wind changes direction, so does the feather. There is flow and lightness. The feather adjusts its course with the wind. There are no expectations, just the feather and the air connecting in the moment. Be like a feather right now and connect with the present moment. Allow thoughts to flow like the wind. Don't dwell; let everything pass. Feel the lightness.

April 26

THE WATER AND THE MOON have an intuitive
connection. It is a powerful process to set intentions
under the moonlight when you are near water. Water is
malleable and absorbs the energy we emit. Since our
bodies are mostly made of water, we are susceptible
to the energy of the moon and that of others. Imagine
floating on your back under the moonlight. As you feel
the water support you and the moon's light, visualize your
intention and offer appreciation for that single moment.

April 27

I ACCEPT WHERE I AM IN MY LIFE. There are no
mistakes, just lessons I have learned. My path has been
forged through perseverance. When I stumble, I get
back up. I accept the trials that have come my way. My
life is rich with experience and I smile because I have
overcome and learned. I offer acceptance to others
because they too are on their own unique path. I do not
know where they are going, but I can send love and
acceptance from my soul to theirs.

April 28

A SEED NEEDS SOIL to grow in and water to make its casing malleable to set forth roots and seedlings. Without water and the warmth from the soil, a seed would not thrive. It needs attention and care. We have seeds in our lives that need attention and care. Some we forget or ignore and they fail to thrive. Tend to those seeds and allow roots to grow. Encourage growth and watch beauty unfold.

———

April 29

AN EMPTY SPACE IS ready to be filled. Anything can happen in this space. Possibilities are seeds in which experience can grow and thrive. Empty does not necessarily mean barren or void. Emptiness can be an opening, a clearing for something new. When something is removed and a space is created, think about the beauty that can replace what once was. Be open, not empty. Use this opportunity for stillness and allow the answer to present itself.

April 30

A GARDEN THAT HAS BEEN neglected has hardened soil, dead plants, and overgrown weeds. A beautiful garden can grow again. Breaking up the dry, cracked ground and removing the dead plants and weeds is just the first step. Our hearts and souls are like gardens. If we neglect them, care needs to occur. Break the hardness up with love and kindness. Find the dead growth and let go. Pull the weeds that hold you back. Growth is on its way.

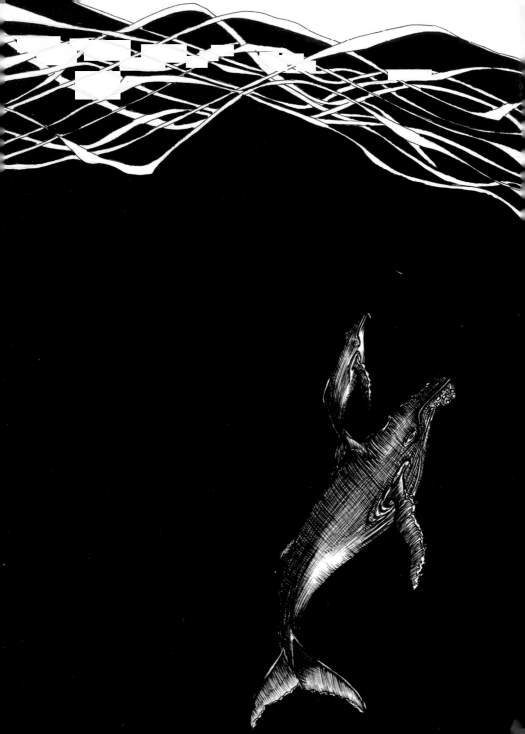

May 1

If you can't sleep, then get up and do something
instead of lying there worrying. It's the worry that gets you,
not the lack of sleep.

—DALE CARNEGIE

RESTLESS NIGHTS CAN ROB US of sleep and fill us
with stress. When restlessness occurs, write down what
is worrying you to remove the thought from actively
working in your mind. After you have recorded these
thoughts, let them go. Breathe in calmness instead of
worry and drift back to sleep.

May 2

FEELINGS ARE LIKE the waves of the ocean: they rise and fall. It is important to be present during each wave and to go with the flow instead of resisting. If a particularly heavy feeling arises, imagine a surfboard diving into it and coming out on the other side. A wave can feel deep and over our head for a moment, but on the other side is breath and calm. Be in the moment, breathe, and allow the heaviness to pass.

———

May 3

BENEATH THE SURFACE of the ocean live many creatures seen and unseen. Some come up to display their beauty and others stay in the depths, yet they are thriving. Each of us has an inner life that can thrive beyond what we project outwardly. To cultivate this, we need to allow moments of stillness in our lives like the depths of the sea. Although the ocean waves swell and break above the surface, below there is an inner stillness where a rich inner life thrives.

May 4

INSIDE EACH OF US IS a strain of wildness that we tame without even knowing it. Keeping the wildness alive inside of us takes less work than restraining it. Moments of pleasure, whether simple or complex, can remind us of our inner nature. What have you been taming in your life that is yearning to come out? Have you been stifling your inner animal for the sake of appearances? Take a moment to connect with your inner wildness. Breathe into your innate primal energy.

May 5

ONCE A YEAR, in the driest environment, a yucca shoots up to the sky and blooms brightly. Its yellow and white blooms breathe energy, color, and vibrancy into the desert landscape. Yuccas show that even in a harsh, parched environment, blooming is possible. If you are going through a particularly difficult time, find an opportunity to reach up and thrive. Being mindful of the pain and allowing growth to take place creates resilience. Resilience breeds strength, which moves us forward.

May 6

WHEN OUR MOST BASIC NEEDS go unmet, we feel unbalanced. It is difficult to unearth ourselves from the rubble of self-defeating thoughts, but it is possible by practicing gratitude and contentment. Even when we feel as if our most basic needs are not met, if you look deeper, you will recognize abundance in your life. Think about three positive things that happened today. No matter how small they are, they are pockets of abundance.

May 7

OUR INNER LIGHTS ARE beacons that attract things to our lives. When we allow outside influences to affect our ability to shine, we may believe that our lights are dimmer than they actually are. But the light still shines. The only thing that can affect our lights are our thoughts and how we perceive ourselves. If we allow another person's thoughts or opinions to contribute to our self-doubt, our lights dim. Take inventory of your thoughts, notice where you are doubting yourself, and shine love into that space.

May 8

THE STORIES WE TELL ourselves have the ability to uplift us or bring us down. Our thoughts determine positive or negative energy that take its course throughout our bodies. Our bodies have seven energy centers beginning at the base of our spine. To balance our root chakra, we can imagine a warm red light emanating from our lower spine outward. Breathe gratitude and abundant thoughts into this light. Know that the universe will meet every need. Let go of control and open up to receiving all the good that is on its way to you.

May 9

SPEAKING OUR TRUTH COMES from a place of courage. At times we must say uncomfortable things, and when left unsaid, our throat chakra can become blocked. When we come from a place of love, even the most difficult conversations can take place. Allow peace to surface. Breathe in a calm turquoise light. Allow the light to cover your throat and vocal cords. Imagine it washing away all the fear and creating a pathway for your words to make their way out.

May 10

WHEN THERE IS AN emotional weakness, especially
one surrounding our primal and creative natures, the
sacral chakra becomes imbalanced. This energy center is
where we physically and spiritually give birth. It is where
creation resides. A balanced center feels innovative
and attractive. Imagine a vibrant orange light emanating
from below your navel. Use this light to attract beautiful,
astonishing ideas and love to you. Create something
beautiful, physically and spiritually.

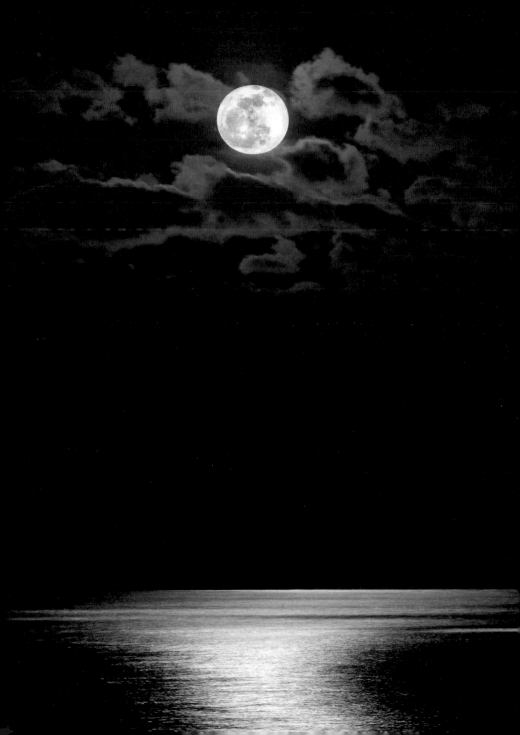

May 11

WORRY AND ANXIETY ARE symptoms of our solar plexus chakra being out of balance. Located right above the navel, this energy center is where our self-confidence and respect live. To doubt ourselves is to deplete our power. Imagine a bright yellow light shooting from your center, where your intuition lies. Feel this light pulling the self-doubt to the surface and ridding your body of self-defeating thoughts. Allow the light to attract confidence and optimism in that space.

May 12

THERE IS SO MUCH POWER in our heart centers, where love resides. When we are balanced, we exude generosity, love, and compassion. When we deny these key functions of the heart, jealousy, bitterness, and fear take their place. The universe provides an example of unconditional love. When we strive to offer this to ourselves and others, our love and compassion grow. Visualize a beautiful green light shining from your heart outward, first surrounding yourself and then others. Allow the light to embrace all things.

May 13

MAY'S FLOWER MOON: Growth and blossoming are taking place all around. Sprouts have become stalks and roots continue to deepen. Blossoms have become flowers and trees start to bear fruit. What is emerging in your life right now? Is there any extra pruning or weeding that you need to do? Give your intentions room to develop. Offer gratitude for the blossoms and weeds in your life. Blossoms offer growth and weeds offer lessons; both are required for wisdom to take root.

———

May 14

Make the most of yourself by fanning the tiny, inner sparks of possibility into flames of achievement.

—GOLDA MEIR

A SPARK CAN IGNITE a forest fire, depending on the fuel available. When something sparks inside our souls, we can fan the flames with desire and determination. With just a little effort, our passions can become actualized dreams. Allow these sparks to help you achieve great things by fanning the flames of your dreams.

May 15

FOCUSING CAN BE DIFFICULT, and we can become distracted going from one thought to another. Our brow chakra is located on the forehead, between our eyes. It is our third eye, where our wisdom and intuitive thoughts are born. When we are focused, we are able to trust our thoughts and tap into our inner wisdom with ease. See a deep blue light shining steadily and calmly from this center inward. Focus on this steady light and feel centered.

———

May 16

OUR DIVINE WISDOM AND LIGHT reside just above our heads, connecting us to the universal force and to all beings. We understand that we are not alone and find peace in this oneness. Open up to this higher knowledge by seeing a purple light, like a crown, emanating from the top of your head and rising upward. Reach for this connection to the divine. Ask for help; accept this peace.

May 17

SOME DECISIONS ARE difficult to make. We can go back and forth with pros and cons and never reach a solution. Deep inside each one of us resides intuition. To tap into our inner guide, we must find stillness. In stillness we can ask for answers and then listen to what our intuition has to say. Without excess noise, we can hear our soul. Some feel it in their gut, others their heart. Take a moment to locate your truth center and connect within.

———

May 18

WHAT WE EAT is important to our sleep and daily rhythms. Nutrition plays a role in our sleep patterns as well as our overall health. Eating is an energy exchange between our bodies and the plant or animal. If we nourish ourselves with good energy, we absorb that energy. The same is true with bad foods that emit a lower energy frequency. Offer appreciation each time you eat and at the end of every day for the nourishment you received.

May 19

WAITING TRIES OUR PATIENCE; every wait has a
lesson and expectations create longing. But as we wait,
patience is building and we can find space to connect
inwardly. Use moments of waiting for contemplation,
gratitude, and meditation. Connect with your breath
and find your center. If you are waiting for something
right now, visualize the outcome and be grateful for this
momentary pause.

May 20

THROUGH THE CRACKS in a sidewalk, weeds can find light. The heavy weight of concrete does not deter them from finding their way into the sunlight. To grow like a weed is to survive. Even if you feel a heavy emotional weight persisting, you are still growing. Reach for the sunlight. Find your way from beneath the weight and push through. Perseverance will find the place where light shines. Through it, you will grow and emerge.

———

May 21

A SCAR REMAINS long after an injury heals. Scars are physical reminders of survival and healing. Emotional scars can also linger and create phantom memories that may emerge from time to time. Scars do not need to be dwelled upon, but can serve as tokens of growth and resilience. The memories need not be a hindrance. Scars create a unique landscape in our hearts and souls that lead the way to restoration.

May 22

FORGIVENESS FREES OUR SOULS from bitterness and resentment. When we forgive, we offer grace and love to ourselves as well as the other people involved. Where there is grace, love and forgiveness grow; darkness cannot thrive. Gifts are given without expectation of something in return, so forgive no matter what. Freedom comes when our hearts soften with forgiveness. There is no need to hold on to the pain. If you have need of forgiveness in your life, start the healing process today.

May 23

FEELINGS OF DEFEAT create despair, which can be difficult to let go of. To overcome self-defeat, be your own inner hero. Write down the thoughts that are cultivating defeats, and then rewrite the narrative from a more compassionate point of view. Stop the negative thought loop by creating a positive spin. Reroute the thoughts and tell fear to move aside. When fear and defeat speak, respond with compassion and love.

May 24

"For my own part, I declare I know nothing whatever about it but to look at the stars always makes me dream."

—VINCENT VAN GOGH

IF YOU COULD HAVE any dream come true, what would it be? The stars are out right now. It's the perfect time for dreaming. As you fall asleep, think about your perfect dream coming true. Picture what it looks like and let your dreams take care of the rest.

———

May 25

If the stars should appear one night in a thousand years, how would men believe and adore; and preserve for many generations the remembrance of the city of God which had been shown! But every night come out these envoys of beauty, and light the universe with their admonishing smile.

—RALPH WALDO EMERSON

NO MATTER WHAT HAPPENS in the universe, the stars continue to shine. For millennia, they have twinkled in the sky. Contemplate this amazing feat as you drift off to sleep.

May 26

OUR DREAMS ARE POWERFUL and create an energy exchange between our brain and the universe. When we believe in our dreams manifesting, we intentionally set the stage for dreams to actualize. A dream is just the beginning: a spark. From this spark, wonderful things can take place. Believe in your dreams. Embrace them and see where they lead. Nothing is too big if you have trust.

———

May 27

IF WE BELIEVE IN THE POWER of our dreams, we can manifest what we desire. Be patient. The universe Is at work. Think about some of the things you hoped for a few years ago. Remember the waiting and wondering that occurred. Notice what has transpired since then. Be grateful for the gifts and also for what is yet to come.

May 28

Everyone is a moon, and has a dark side
which he never shows to anybody."
—MARK TWAIN

OUR DARK SIDE DOES NOT necessarily need to be hidden. Darkness can exist where stillness resides. We can look inward without the influence of others and get in touch with our higher selves. Our souls and the universe communicate in stillness. Find time every day to foster this still place where the influence of others is void.

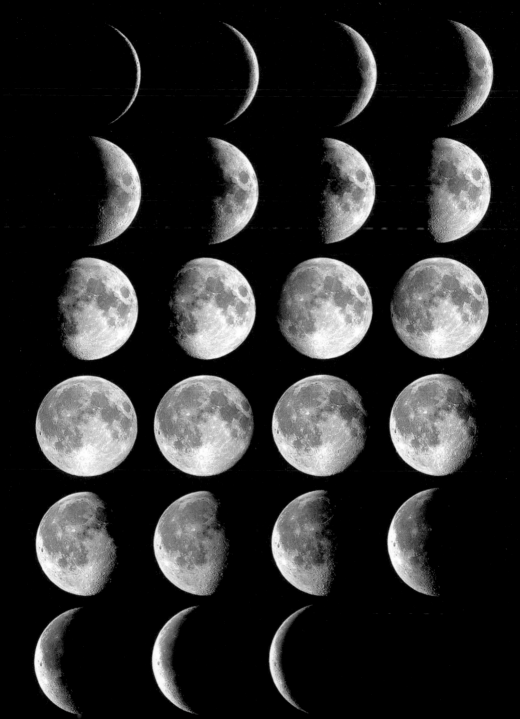

May 29

WHAT MAKES YOUR SOUL EXPAND? It may be beauty that brings about a long stare or the moments of awe and wonder that leave you speechless. Many amazing things can connect us to creation. When moments of expansion arise, breathe deeply into the moment and be grateful for the opportunity to witness wonder.

————

May 30

Trust in dreams, for in them is hidden the gate to eternity.
—KHALIL GIBRAN

DEEP IN OUR SLEEP, our conscious mind makes way for the subconscious to awaken. For years, people have interpreted their dreams and found connections that are not as obvious during waking hours. Keep a journal by your bed and chronicle your dreams upon awakening. Connect with your dreams and understand their meanings. See if there are patterns or symbols that are asking for attention. Trust and open your mind to their messages.

May 31

ABUNDANCE IS ALL AROUND. Even in the lean times, if we look closely, abundance abounds. The universe is constantly providing for our needs and our prayers should not be only requests, but also gratitude. When your joy is full and the day is done, remember to pray with gratefulness for the abundance in your life.

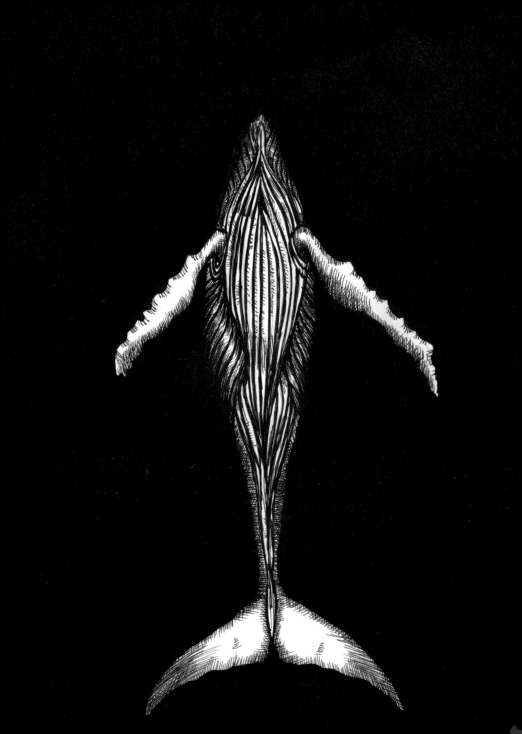

June 1

Do not dwell in the past, do not dream of the future,
concentrate the mind on the present moment.

—BUDDHA

THE PAST WAS ONCE THE PRESENT, and at that time
it was important. When we dwell on the past, we ignore
the wonderful things that are happening right before
our eyes. The past plays a significant part in our lives
and development. Presence does not ignore the past; it
merely refocuses attention on what is right in front of us.

June 2

A GALAXY WITHIN OUR SPIRITS connects us to one another. Just like the stars in a galaxy, we too interconnect. Getting in touch with our spirit and acknowledging the mystery that is the divine awakens a bond. We have more similarities than meet the eye. As we live, we connect. When we die, we return to the land, sea, and air. We do not end; we continue to connect.

———

June 3

NATURE BRINGS US BACK to our most basic selves. Everything is connected and is part of a cyclical process. In nature we can connect to a wildness that everyday life tames. Our connection to our primal side motivates our drive and survival. Spend time in nature this week. Connect with your inner nature. Allow freedom to take root and reconnect with the divine.

June 4

WHEN WE CHASE THINGS, they can seem perpetually just out of reach. There is an illusion of control in the chase. But the more we try to control, the less control we actually have. When we let things go, what we are searching for has the freedom to appear or even return to us.

———

June 5

WHEN THE SEAS OF LIFE seem choppy, this is not the time to retreat and hide. In the eye of the storm, a skilled sailor is most alert, sailing the ship through it instead of freezing in fear. Grab hold of the helm and navigate through the storm to calmer waters. The calm comes before and after a storm. Instincts are stronger and more attuned after going through a storm.

June 6

GROWTH IS A PAINFUL PROCESS that often brings a great sense of relief when completed. Think about a time when you went through a period of growth. Think about who you were before, during, and after that time. Give thanks for the grace you experienced during the transition and know that with each new growth a beautiful blossom appears.

———

June 7

GRATITUDE IS THE MOST IMPORTANT prayer of the day. Offering gratitude expresses the acknowledgment of the beautiful things in life. The ability to find things to be grateful for during difficult times strengthens spiritual muscles and attracts more things we can be grateful for in our lives. Take a moment to reflect on the day and express gratitude for the bright spots and opportunities for growth.

June 8

The truth dazzles gradually, or else the world would be blind.
—EMILY DICKINSON

HAVING IMMEDIATE ANSWERS would be wonderful because there would be no room for ambiguity. But if the truth were revealed and all were known, there would be no room for wonder. Allow the spaces of not knowing to create a beautiful anticipation of truth. Even there, magic and wonder can be found. Embrace the unknown with the hope of being dazzled.

June 9

OUR PERSPECTIVES CREATE our reality. If we tend to focus on outside factors, we may find ourselves in a dream state. This is not necessarily a bad place to be, but we need to make sure that we move forward. When we look inward, we can hear the still, small voice the universe provides. The soul awakens only when we gaze inward.

June 10

OUR ESSENCE REMAINS because our souls continue even after our bodies die. When a star shoots through the sky, its particles get absorbed back into the universe. Everything is interconnected and our essences are universal. Pay attention to how things are connected and appreciate the presence of all things.

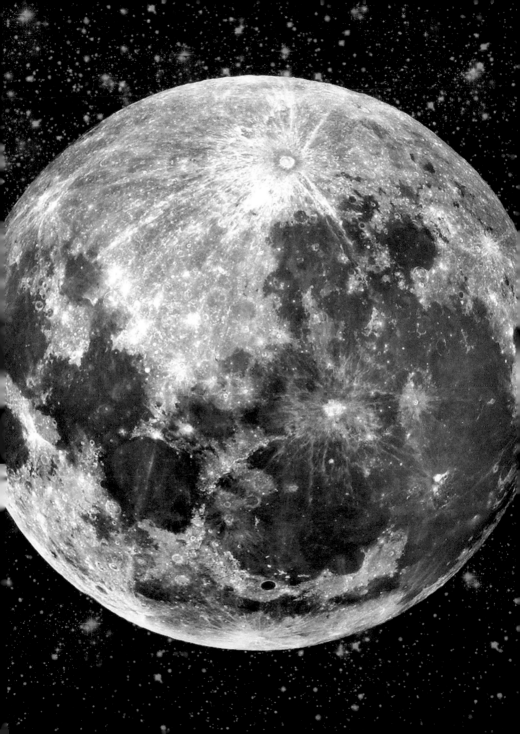

June 11

AN ARTIST'S HANDS MOLD a pot from a lump of clay. With care, each turn of the wheel gets the clay closer to the potter's vision. Afterwards, the artist puts the pot into a kiln. Through shaping and fire, a beautiful creation emerges from a lump of clay. Sometimes we need fire to enhance our beauty. Remember that in the end, we can emerge as beautiful vessels if we are malleable like clay.

———

June 12

HOW GOOD DOES IT FEEL when someone says "thank you"? Genuine appreciation validates our efforts and creates a reciprocal bond of gratitude. Offering appreciation from the heart extends gratitude and fulfills an inner craving we all have. Make a point to extend appreciation to at least one person this week. This practice will brighten your life as well as theirs.

June 13

JUNE'S STRAWBERRY MOON: Ripening berries fill the night air with a sweet aroma. As the air is becoming warmer, plants and trees offer their sweetness. What sweetness can you offer right now? Is there a difficult situation that you could soften with the harmony that sweetness can provide? Perhaps there is fruit in your life that is ripening and maturing. Growth is an evolution. As you drift off to sleep tonight, contemplate where in your life you can infuse kindness and the wisdom of growth.

———

June 14

The darker the night, the brighter the stars,
the deeper the grief, the closer is God!
—FYODOR DOSTOYEVSKY

GRIEF PERMEATES OUR SOULS like nothing else. It takes time to heal from the pain and sorrow of loss. Allow the awareness that something greater is holding on to you and can be a source of comfort during periods of grief. Draw near to this source and allow it to be the light during dark times.

June 15

WHAT DID YOU THINK ABOUT ALL DAY? Think about any patterns that recur. Are your thoughts fixated repeatedly on the same things? If there is something you want or are striving to become, spend some time visualizing that. Direct your thoughts toward the things you want rather than the things you do not want. Our thoughts control our focus.

———

June 16

PEACE COMES FROM WITHIN. Understanding comes from lessons learned. During times of unease, know that a new understanding is forming. The process is continuous, fluid, and ever changing. It is important to stay open and allow each experience to flow as needed. Search for the meaning in stillness. There, peace will sprout.

June 17

WHAT MESSAGE DOES your life convey? Even if we think no one is watching, there is an audience. Even the way we treat strangers communicates this message. What we give, we receive. What would you like to receive in life? Identify what you would like your message to be, as well as what you would like to receive. Find where your life aligns and notice where you need to make adjustments. Honor yourself and others with your message.

———

June 18

Somewhere, something incredible is waiting to be known.
—CARL SAGAN

WE MAY NOT KNOW what the future holds, but possibility and wonder are waiting to be discovered. Don't stop searching for the beauty in life. Always look for ways to find the incredible and lovely in every day. You can always discover something, whether it is external or internal. When you identify the wonder of the day, offer genuine gratitude.

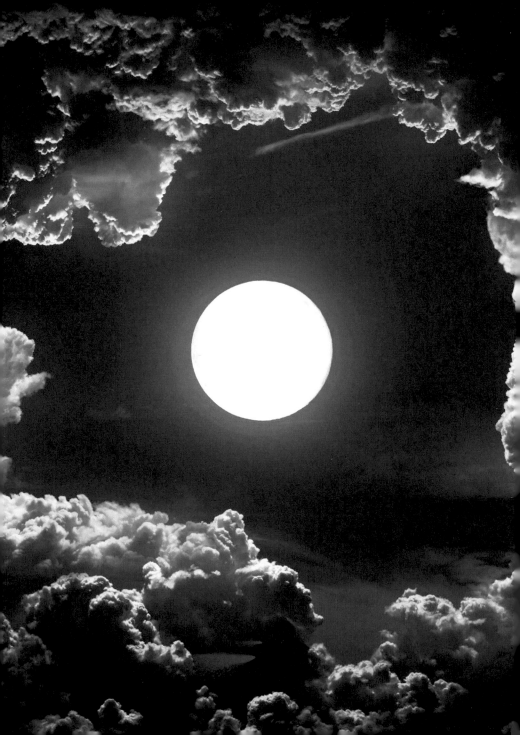

June 19

PLEASURE LIES IN DISCOVERY. Not knowing creates an anticipatory excitement that can fuel the search and bring even greater joy in finding. If you are searching for something, find the joy in the unknown. Embrace the pursuit and allow the anticipation to build. After the wait your answer will feel like a reward, like buried treasure.

June 20

WHEN WE LOOK BACK on our lives, we will not remember the little things that vex us. We will laugh at how preoccupied we were with such inconsequential issues. Why let them take up our time now? Tonight, think about which problems you might be giving more power than they deserve. Cast those tiny worries from your mind, and sleep soundly without them.

———

June 21

WAITING IS DIFFICULT, especially when what you are anticipating feels important. Rest in knowing that the universe unfolds at just the right time. When you feel the pang of longing, breathe into the peace that everything is being taken care of. Clarity is on its way.

June 22

WHEN AMAZING THINGS HAPPEN, the result can feel overwhelming. After long waits or striving for results, victory can catch us off guard. Revel in your success. Feel the pride that comes from working hard and creating desired results. The most important thing is to offer gratitude for the delivery of your manifestation. Some things are meant to feel this good.

June 23

*Live the full life of the mind, exhilarated by new ideas,
intoxicated by the Romance of the Unusual.*

—ERNEST HEMINGWAY

THE UNKNOWN HAS A SENSE of romance and wonder tied to it. Every day we have a chance to fill our minds with new, exciting information that can awaken curiosity and knowledge in our minds. Take time each day to receive something new. Allow wonder to take place and romance to grow from the unknown.

June 24

WHEN CLOUDS PART and the sky opens up, rain falls, refreshing rivers, lakes, and plants. Soon after the rain falls, the sun's light shines down, illuminating what was once parched and dry. When we allow our hearts to open and awaken to love, our souls are refreshed and light shines through us. We can build and mend relationships when we keep our hearts open and let the light of love come in.

———

June 25

With freedom, books, flowers and the moon,
who could not be happy?
—OSCAR WILDE

LIFE HAS MANY SIMPLE PLEASURES. Appreciation for them breeds happiness and contentment. The moon and stars come out every night to display their brilliance after millennia. For our short time on Earth, we too should shine and be grateful for each moment and the daily gifts it gives us. Look around; sources of happiness are all around us.

June 26

FOR A WAVE TO SWELL, energy needs to travel across the ocean at just the right time. It rises and falls. A flower that starts from a seed takes time to spout, bud, and blossom. Babies need time to develop before birth. Nature displays patience and beauty without complaint. If you are waiting for something to come along, think about how some of the most beautiful things take their precious time.

June 27

VISUALIZATION CAN AID in seeing what we really want, where we want to go, and who we want to be. When the eyes are shut, we allow the brain to create the images for us. The things we hope for, think about, and are determined to create have room to express themselves in this space. For a few moments, close your eyes and visualize an outcome you desire. See it as if it is happening right before you.

June 28

BEING CONTENT COMES from gratitude for everything just as it is. Practicing gratitude attracts more things to be grateful for. The key is to find contentment and happiness right where we are. If you are working toward something, be grateful for the ability to do the work, the time you have to get the job done, and the drive to achieve something great.

———

June 29

Be in love with your life every detail of it.
—JACK KEROUAC

TO LOVE SOMETHING DOES not mean that it is lovable only when it is perfect. The imperfections can draw us closer and intrigue us. Life has times that are less than ideal. Going through the valleys creates depth and appreciation for our journey, as well as the journey of others. Embrace every moment and find the glimmer of love in difficult times. These times lead to a sense of joy when they pass.

June 30

WHAT WAS THE MOST beautiful thing you saw today?
Take a moment to reflect on the beauty you beheld. Think
about how it made you feel. In that moment, you found
the joy of being present and allowed beauty to stop you in
your tracks. Look for beauty every day. Allow time to stand
still in the face of beauty, even if only for a moment.

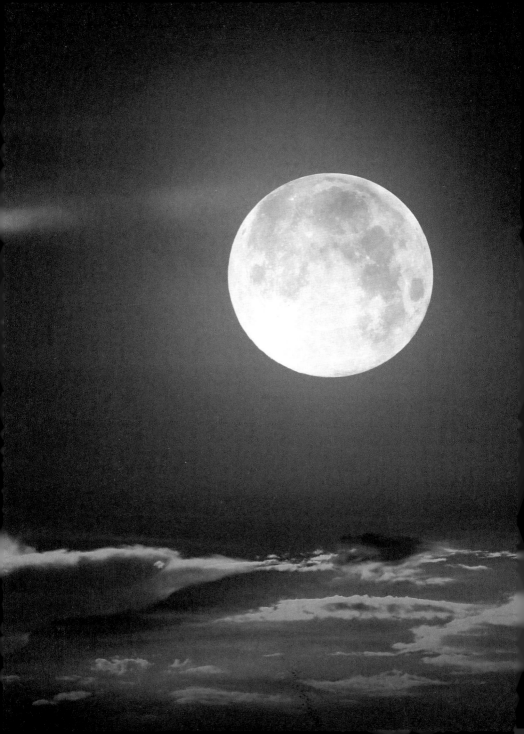

July 1

A STILL MIND IS QUIET despite the endless loop
of everyday noise. In stillness, answers are revealed
and breath finds the rhythm of the heart. Letting go
of thoughts and surrendering into stillness creates the
space for revelations and understanding. Getting in sync
with the universe can happen when we open our minds
in quiet and listen to the voice within.

July 2

WAITING FOR ANSWERS can make us anxious and impatient. In the space of waiting is the opportunity to be blank and open. Patience allows; anxiety pushes. Stay open and allow great things to come your way. Don't force or try to control them. Everything happens at just the right time. Rest in knowing that timing is everything.

———

July 3

*Jump, and you will find out how to unfold
your wings as you fall.*

—RAY BRADBURY

WE CAN TRY TO PLAN every detail of our lives, but something can always get in our way. Taking risks requires faith and trusting that you have the resources to overcome obstacles. You can always find ways to gather what you need along the way. But the outcome will never be known unless you take that first step. Leap—and trust that the universe has your needs covered.

July 4

FAITH IS TRUSTING IN THINGS we cannot see,
things that are grounded in the soul. When our minds
take over, our faith wavers and we find excuses as to
why the unknown will not work or is scary. Fear thrives
in a faithless environment. But faith challenges fear. It is
more powerful—and when faith happens, miracles occur.

——————

July 5

EXPANSION GENERATES the blossom from the
bud and the breath from our lungs. Opening our eyes
to beauty expands our connection to the creator, to
ourselves, and to others. We are all connected; see the
wonder in every little thing.

July 6

THE DEEPEST CONNECTIONS COME from within our souls. To harness our courage, we create unbounded freedom. In this space, our light illuminates our minds to experiences beyond our comprehension. The divine hears your every wish, and this illustrates that your soul connects you to something grander than the physical realm.

———

July 7

Grief can be the garden of compassion. If you keep your heart open through everything, your pain can become your greatest ally in your life's search for love and wisdom.

—RUMI

OUR EMOTIONS CREATE our experiences. When we choose to grow in response to our sorrows, we plant seeds of love and wisdom within our souls. Although our sorrows may not feel light, our tears are watering the seeds we choose to plant.

July 8

DARKNESS DOES NOT necessarily hinder movement. We can find a path when we choose to stay still and find insight. In times of darkness, stillness can produce a light within as a guide. With this light, darkness has no room to overbear. It can reflect the glow of inner light and become the stage for enlightenment.

———

July 9

DREAMS DO NOT LIVE without our thoughts and emotions. We are the dream makers and anything is possible. Whatever you desire, reach for it and visualize the dream. Set your attention on great things and not just on why or how it will happen. Choose to reach.

July 10

"And all the loveliest things there be
Come simply, so it seems to me."

—EDNA ST. VINCENT MILLAY

THE MOON RISES AS ALWAYS, leaving this day behind as it steadily climbs into the night sky. The past is gone, and another night, another moonrise, is all that matters. As the day passes into night, feel the worries of the day evaporate out of you. Focus on the simple stillness of this moment, when everything in the world is at peace.

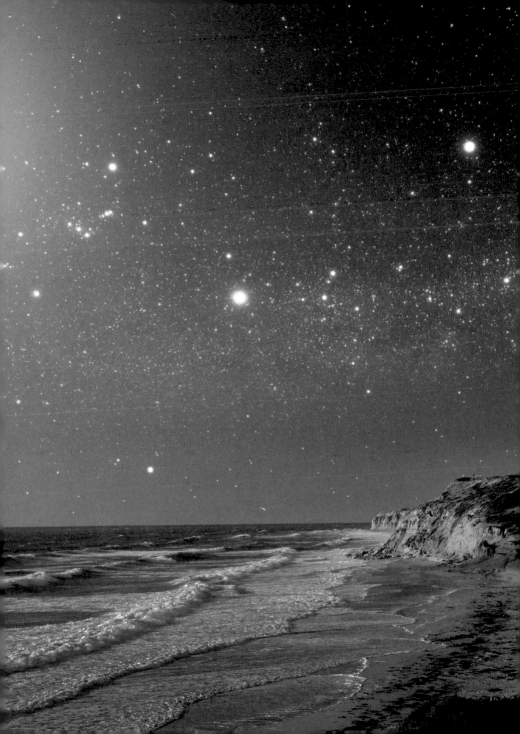

July 11

The big question is whether you are going to be
able to say a hearty yes to your adventure.
—JOSEPH CAMPBELL

WE ARE NOT MEANT to live a mundane existence. We have a choice to explore the amazing world in which we live. Whether they are local, national, or beyond, amazing things are all around us. Saying yes every day to finding the adventure in life brings variety and wonder. Your next adventure may be right around the corner or on the other side of the world. Just show up and be willing to explore.

———

July 12

NEVER STOP GIVING THANKS. Every moment, we have something to be grateful for. The lungs we breathe with, the home where we live, the sun that shines and makes everything grow. These are just a few of the simple things that occur every day. When we dig deeper, the well of gratitude overflows. There is so much to be grateful for.

July 13

JULY'S THUNDER MOON: Thunderstorms roar across
the sky as warm air builds up and lightning strikes through
the clouds. When something is building up in your life, look
for ways to release the pressure. Thunder grabs attention.
Is there an area in your life that needs attention? Use this
time to reflect on any changes you need to make. Allow
whatever needs to be released to fall away. Only then can
you make room for what is yet to be.

July 14

IN RELATIONSHIPS, OUR GOAL SHOULD BE to nurture
each other, creating a beautiful garden full of love. When
the need to control arises, question the fear driving that
need. Communicate in love and allow fear to subside.
Dominance does not create the room for growth; it leads
to contraction. Notice any lingering fear and breathe love
into that space.

July 15

It takes courage to grow up and become who you really are.
—E. E. CUMMINGS

WHEN WE BECOME COMPLACENT in our comfort zone, we are not tapping into our full potential. It can be scary to go after our desires. There is fear of failure and rejection that lingers before courage takes place. But to truly actualize your potential, you must harness your bravery to move forward, leaving complacency behind.

July 16

THUNDER SOUNDS HIGH above the mountains. Various shades of gray fill the sky, which turns darker as the moments pass. Soon the heavens open up and a veil of rain pours down, releasing built-up pressure. The ground becomes saturated. As quickly as it began, the storm passes and steam rises from the warm earth. Life can feel chaotic and out of control in the middle of life's storms, but they always pass. Let the pressure release and allow the rain to fall.

July 17

LIVING IN THE PAST ALLOWS yearning to take hold of our hearts. We may reference supposed glory days as a standard, but then we forget that in fact the greatest things lie ahead of us. Focus on the present moment instead of ruminating on the past or projecting into the future. What we create right here, right now, molds what is next. Seize this moment while having gratitude for the past.

July 18

WHEN NIGHT FALLS, jasmine reveals its intoxicating fragrance. The blooms open under the moonlight to emit a sweet aroma that is pleasing and memorable. During the day, many flowers display their beauty under the sun, but jasmine patiently waits until the other blooms go to sleep. This is a reminder that we too can showcase our beauty after patiently waiting. In darkness, we can still radiate beauty.

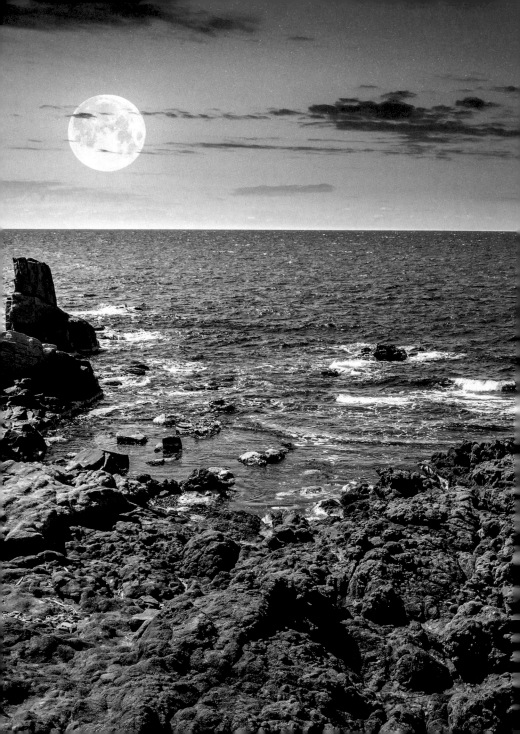

July 19

"One should not spoil what is present by desiring
what is absent, but rather reason out that these things
too were among those we might have prayed for."

—EPICURUS

TAKE A MOMENT TO RECOGNIZE all the gifts life has
delivered. Remember the times when you yearned for
these things. Be thankful for those dreams and requests
that came to fruition and notice that the universe hears
your every desire. If you are waiting for something, know
that in time, the answer will be revealed.

July 20

TIMING IS EVERYTHING when you are waiting for things to happen. In time, your answer will come. The space in between is a lovely place to reflect, be grateful, and redirect your focus if needed. Just like a river that eventually makes it to the ocean, your desires find their way to fruition. Trust the timing and know that when you are ready, the outcome will appear.

———

July 21

IF LIFE WERE A CONSTANT barrage of overwhelming stimuli, we would become numb to awe. The secret is to find joy in simple things. Daily meals and clean drinking water are just as amazing as something out of the ordinary. Find time to celebrate life's simplicities; this will make room for more awe.

July 22

TRUE FREEDOM LIES IN the ability to be brave and take the leap into the life you are meant to live. It can be scary to leap without knowing what the outcome may be. Fear can cloud the ability to see the beauty of truly letting go. Taking bold moves creates bold momentum. If you have been dreaming of doing something, visualize the outcome and feel bravery as you drift toward sleep.

July 23

Wonder is the beginning of wisdom.
—ARISTOTLE

A CHILD IS FULL OF WONDER and learns from exploring the unknown. Being able to see things with fresh eyes and perspective can open our minds to deeper wisdom. Try looking at a familiar situation from a different viewpoint. See if you can gain any new wisdom by opening your mind to the situation a little more.

July 24

*The world is full of magic things patiently
waiting for our wits to grow sharper.*

—EDEN PHILLPOTTS

TO SEE ALL OF THE WONDER the world has to offer,
we must get in touch with the soul of things. Connecting
at a deeper level involves looking past the surface and
practicing presence. Our breath can bring us into the
moment, allowing distractions to fall away. Set the intention
to connect and unveil what lies below the surface.

———

July 25

A BLINDFOLD MAY HINDER the ability to see what is
right before us, but it does not keep us from seeing. If
we choose to keep our eyes shielded, we can ignore the
view, but not what is happening. Eventually, we must
face every truth. Avoidance does not make things go
away. Through avoidance, we may craft stories that skew
the truth. Seek the truth, open your eyes, and be present
with what is happening right now.

July 26

SLEEP IS NOT INSTANTANEOUS. We cannot expect to be busy and preoccupied right before we go to sleep. We must ease ourselves into calm and peace, so as not to muddy it with half-finished tasks and half-thought ideas. Tonight, ease into bed one step at a time. Take a moment to meditate and clear your mind of nagging cares. Then, get ready for sleep.

July 27

EROSION REVEALS THE LAYERS of a cliff. The ocean spends years pounding against the jagged edge of the earth, trying to show its power. In time, the cliff submits and another layer is revealed. The cliff softens and at times crumbles into the powerful waves of the sea. No matter how much erosion occurs, beauty remains where a tall cliff once stood. The same can be said about the walls we build around our hearts. Allow the love and forgiveness of others to wear down the walls and reveal something beautiful.

July 28

AFTER THE AIR COOLS in the desert, a rattlesnake makes its way out from under a rock. It slithers across the ground feeling the contrast of the cool air and the warmth left on the ground from the day's hot sun. Instinct tells the snake when to go out, explore, and seek food. If left alone, the snake does not feel threatened, nor does it strike. When balanced, we follow our natural instincts; we don't feel the need to react or harm.

———

July 29

A RUNNER GOES THROUGH PAIN to win a race. After months of muscle tears, blisters, and shin splints, the body is conditioned for the race. Through the trials and injuries, a runner sees the results of hard work. Glory is found at the finish line, no matter what time is achieved. Through life's trials, remember that there is an end to the pain. Strength is growing. Have faith and trust that all things are working out.

July 30

AS AN EAGLE SOARS, it sees the ground from a higher perspective. Its eyes scan for prey and notices more than when close to the ground. Sometimes we are too close to a situation or outcome to see the big picture. Taking a step back and assessing a situation from a different viewpoint can help create separation. From this vantage point, you can assess and make decisions. A step back can lead to a leap forward.

July 31

WHEN HEALING TAKES PLACE, there is discomfort. A wound heals in layers, whether physical or emotional. In time, the discomfort fades, along with the scar. We need to allow time for our wants to heal and for renewal where the injury occurred. Although we may feel some discomfort, with time, healing will replenish the place where the wound was. Allow the recovery to happen. Develop strength and resilience. Where you once felt great pain, you can become stronger and vibrant.

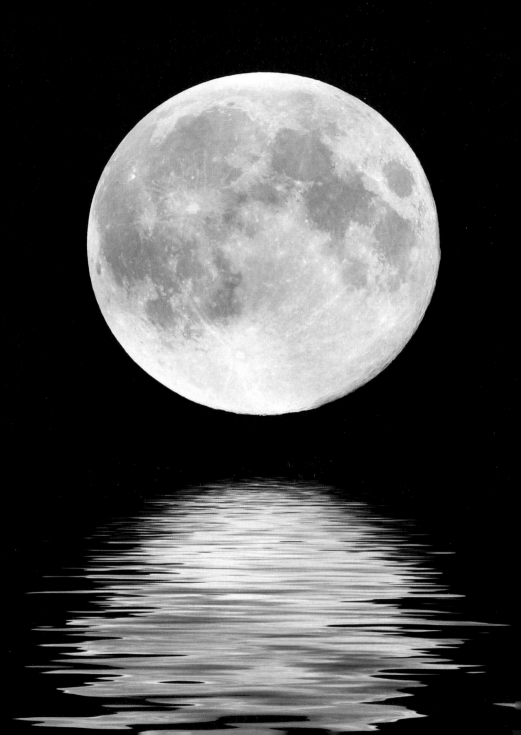

August 1

Synchronicity is an ever present reality for
those who have eyes to see.

—CARL JUNG

COINCIDENCES OCCUR OFTEN and may seem random.
Synchronicity is a beautiful thing when the coincidence
seems meaningful. With an open heart and mind, you can
find meaning and make connections. There is magic within
synchronicity that creates a surge in the soul. Approach
life with open eyes and an open heart, and be ready to see
the magic the universe delivers.

August 2

A DANCER FINDS a focal point while spinning around. Her focus creates balance and grace in her dance. Inner focus creates momentum that helps generate desired results. When our minds spin in a frantic loop, it is easy to lose balance and become thrown off. Finding an inner focal point is key to moving forward. Take a moment to locate an inner focal point. Perhaps it is your breath or your heartbeat. Use this as a guide when life spins.

August 3

I still believe that in spite of everything
people are truly good at heart.
—ANNE FRANK

GOODNESS IS EVERYWHERE. Deep down, we all have needs and desires we wish to be met and validated. Sometimes our goodness is thwarted by negative thoughts and emotions. If you experienced an unpleasant encounter today, offer that person empathy and notice where there may be goodness within. Send that person love and hope that their tomorrow may be better.

August 4

LETTING GO OF THE PAST is a difficult process, but if we held on to each thing we have ever been attached to, the weight would be too much to bear. There is freedom and lightness in releasing what no longer fits into our lives. When old patterns, relationships, and clutter are cleared out, we make space for growth and for new things to enter our lives. Make room for what is to come by releasing your grasp on the past.

———

August 5

SMALL ACTS OF KINDNESS shift energy for the giver and the receiver. Something as simple as a smile or holding a door can turn moods around. It is important to extend kindness to all living things, including ourselves. As the final moments of the day occur, take some time to offer kindness to yourself. Compliment something you accomplished today, or perhaps the way you looked. Embrace yourself with loving-kindness and be grateful for your day.

August 6

WAVES RIPPLE GENTLY along the shore of the bay. The sky turns from soft pastels to deeper, darker hues of the night. Peace and quiet abound. The day is done; all is well. Our thoughts are like the waves, slowly rippling in and out. When we desire peace, we can replace negative thoughts with a simple mantra to coincide with our breath: "I am calm. I am at peace. I am at rest."

August 7

PATIENCE IN THE MIDST of a storm is difficult to cultivate. Anxiety does not create an ideal environment for patience. Therefore, it is even more important to exercise stillness during periods of upheaval. By practicing patience and stillness when it seems near impossible, we develop strength and wisdom. Breathe in the expansive space you create and breathe out the constricting anxiety. All is well. All will be calm soon.

August 8

ENERGY FLOWS FREELY and we get back what we give. If you are feeling particularly light, notice the energy that surrounds you. Pay attention to the energy exchanges that occur. We have the power to change the way we present our energy and can therefore attract what we desire in our lives. When negative thoughts creep up, reframe them and change the energy you ascribe to that thought. Good in, good out.

August 9

THROUGH THE NIGHT SKY, a bat nimbly flies between branches. She navigates the air with sonar, calling out and sensing the objects off which the sound energy bounces. In this way, she navigates the darkness. By sending out our own energy, we can see which parts of our lives are solid, and which parts are only shadows. Send out your gratitude, and take comfort in those things solid enough to return it.

August 10

IN TIMES OF UNCERTAINTY, know that there is a plan. Although we may not have a map, we are on a path where trust and faith take us much farther than doubt and worry do. Try not to become stagnant or stuck. Move forward, even if you take tiny steps. Just as sailors get through the fog using a compass, we have an inner compass: intuition. Tap into it and trust the guidance it offers.

———

August 11

Nothing in life is to be feared. It is only to be understood.
—MARIE CURIE

FEAR CREATES A FALSE SENSE of reality. When we allow fear to take over our thoughts, a loop is created and we begin to believe the worst-case scenario. Instead of falling victim to this thinking, pause and mindfully approach the situation in stillness. Look for understanding. Notice what is truth and what fear is augmenting and distorting. Don't back down. Resolve to understand and grow.

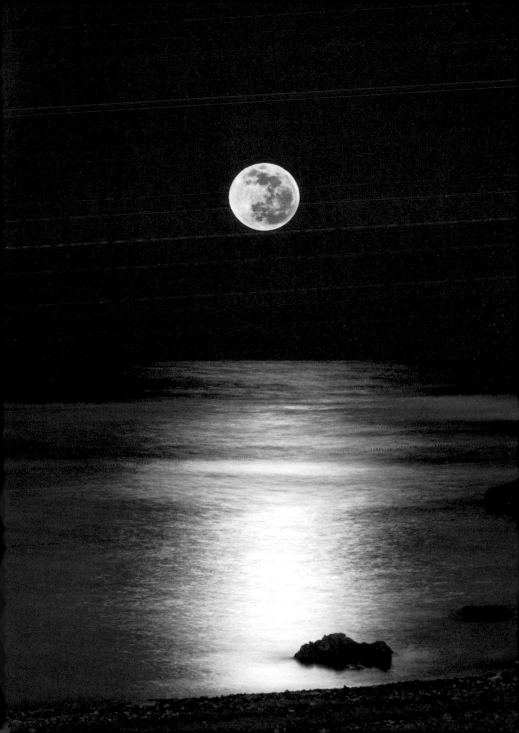

August 12

WE BUILD SAND CASTLES knowing that they will soon wash away. We playfully retrieve water from the ocean to wet the sand. Then, we mold the sand into various shapes, making the structure of the castle. Even though the structure is temporary, we use great care in building it. Nothing in life is permanent, and, like a sand castle, everything will wash away. Take care with anything you set out to achieve. Even temporary things deserve attention and care.

August 13

AUGUST'S STURGEON MOON: This full moon was significant to Native Americans as lakes and rivers filled with fish ready to be caught. Fishing rewards those who are patient. Imagine yourself sitting on the shores of a beautiful lake. The water is calm, your line is cast, and you are still. As you wait for fish to bite, you take in deep breaths, fully present and aware. Nothing needs to happen while you wait. The present moment is all that matters.

August 14

WHEN WE SWIM, coming up for air is a constant process. We fill our lungs so that we can dive back in and envelop ourselves in water. Air and water mix to create a weightless experience; floating becomes effortless. Letting go is essential to floating, trusting the water to hold our weight. When we resist, we begin to sink. Tonight, let go and lie down. Don't resist sleep. Become weightless on your pillow and float into dreamland.

August 15

SHELLS SCATTERED ALONG the beach vary in shape and size. Each one was once a home to a vulnerable creature. Waves reveal deeper layers of the sand where the shells remain. Each wave washes away debris, revealing just a bit more. We can shed the places where we hide our vulnerabilities like the shells along a beach. Open up to connection. Feel the waves of emotion wash away fear and gain strength from the exposure. Vulnerability is beautiful and can lead to deeper connection.

August 16

INVITE PEACE TO ENTER your soul. The day has ended and all of its troubles are over. Take a moment to practice this breathing exercise before you fall asleep: Breathe in peace; breathe out worry. Breathe in peace; breathe out dangling thoughts. Breathe in peace; breathe out stress. Breathe in peace and allow all tension to slowly leave your body, from your head to your toes.

August 17

WITH THE GUIDANCE OF their elders, orcas travel together. These creatures have a strong need for social interaction and thrive as a group. You can see them swimming close to one another in cooperation. Their connections run deep. We all have relationships that require cooperation. Take note of how you can draw closer to develop a deeper connection. When we create the space for others to draw near, connections thrive.

August 18

A CAMPFIRE CRACKLES under the spotlight of the moon. Stars shine as night lingers on. The warmth of the fire offers comfort. Crickets chirp and sounds dim as night fosters slumber. Under a canopy of stars, little things fade away. The grandeur of the universe is there to see if we look up and within. In the final moments of the day, create space for stillness and awe.

———

August 19

DEEP IN THE HEART OF THE OCEAN, whales swim, surrounded by vast amounts of water. They surface to breathe in air before descending below the surface. It is amazing how something so large can move so gracefully and with such ease. Even when we feel as if we are in too deep, it is important to come up for air. Nothing is too big to be resolved. Allow the depths to encourage breathing and restoration.

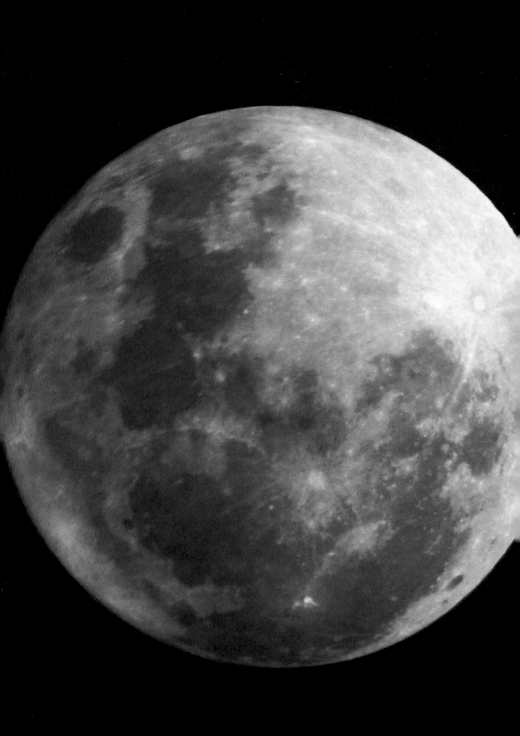

August 20

THE GREATEST GIFT we can offer ourselves is compassion. Many things can and will go wrong. It is important to love ourselves through each mistake and trial. Love and compassion start with the self and can then extend outwardly. Before you go to sleep, do a scan of your body and emotions and find the places where you need love and compassion. Offer yourself these gifts and **settle** into a peaceful sleep.

August 21

CHANGES ARE CONSTANTLY taking place. Consider a caterpillar that begins its life low to the ground and then must create a cocoon. Once encased, the caterpillar must say goodbye to a life that was familiar in order to move on. During the metamorphosis, significant changes take place and a butterfly emerges with the ability to fly. Let whatever needs to happen occur. You are about to fly.

August 22

THE STARS SERVE as a guide at sea. Canoes and great ships alike were led by the positions of stars that still appear. Their illumination and formations have endured for centuries. If the stars can shine and guide many, our inner light can shine and guide as well. All we have to do is find stillness and search for direction. Every night, we have the opportunity to still our minds before we sleep, to calibrate our inner compass. Use this moment to find your direction.

August 23

A MOTHER BIRD PROTECTS her eggs so that development can take place inside the thin shell. Over time, a bird forms within the egg and breaks free. When we experience change, it can feel as if pressure is building. Know that you can break through this pressure when the time is right. Allow the pressure to develop and break free when you feel ready to fly. Release any tension and ease into the change that is occurring.

August 24

EXPECTATIONS CREATE the potential for disappointment. When things don't go the way we expect them to, we may become upset and discouraged. The need to control becomes strong as we try to mold an experience to shape our expectations. Release expectations so that freedom can take place. Letting go of the outcome allows the mind and body to rest. Whatever expectations you may have, release them before you sleep. Create space in your mind for free and peaceful rest.

August 25

The wound is the place where the light enters you.
—RUMI

BROKEN HEARTS HEAL. We heal from the wounds we incur and gain a deeper understanding of ourselves and others. If we choose to allow light to shine through our pain, we can offer inspiration to others who are going through similar pain. Insight, perspective and wisdom will come. Light can permeate where there was once darkness.

August 26

AFTER A STORM PASSES, a rainbow fills the sky. Dark clouds make way for the colorful display, reminding us to count our blessings. Storms can be blessings, as they clear the air and wash away debris. Rains provide much-needed water to replenish the soil. A storm can signify abundance and the rainbow is like a bow on this gift of abundance. The next time you are going through a storm, remember that in the end there is a rainbow of hope.

August 27

A happy life consists not in the absence,
but in the mastery of hardships.

—HELEN KELLER

EACH HARDSHIP IS AN OPPORTUNITY to become
stronger. A gift is present in every difficulty. Think about
times when something was difficult and how it made you
grow in wisdom and strength. Notice where you created
and honed your resilience. Appreciate the knowledge
and competencies that hardship revealed. Life is a series
of lessons. Offer gratitude for each challenge you have
overcome and for the inner power attained.

August 28

GENEROSITY IS A RECIPROCAL GIFT because the
giver not only gives but also receives. When we give
from the heart, we experience a warmth that fills us with
gratitude. In the moment of giving, we can be grateful
for the abundance in our lives and the ability to give—
and we can remember times when we were in need
and received help. We can always find an opportunity
to give. The universe provides us with time, talents, and
resources. Use your gifts to fill a need.

August 29

You must learn to be still in the midst of activity and to be
vibrantly alive in repose.

—INDIRA GANDHI

IN THE MIDST OF STILLNESS, vibrancy is restored.
Finding quiet in chaos allows you to recharge your inner
glow. Learning to be still is a practice that reaps great
rewards. Just like a good night's sleep delivers vitality for
the day ahead, stillness restores mind, body, and soul.
Embrace stillness to shine a little brighter.

August 30

IN THE CENTER OF A MANDALA, peace is created.
The patterns extend outward in a meditative circle. Each
layer is a step closer to peace. A beautiful bloom appears
as the design unfolds. Repetition can soften the mind
into a state of deep rest. Imagine that you are in the
center of the mandala and see each breath extending
outward, surrounding you in a state of peace. Soften into
the peace and make room to rest.

August 31

Love rests on no foundation. It is an endless ocean,
with no beginning or end.

—RUMI

OCEANS RUN DEEP and surround the Earth. Their
borders are invisible as they run into each other,
constantly ebbing and flowing with the cycles of the
moon. Love runs deep and can permeate the soul of
another being. The spaciousness love creates can feel
as vast as the oceans' depths. Let love be fluid. Let the
rising and the falling occur, knowing that love is endless.

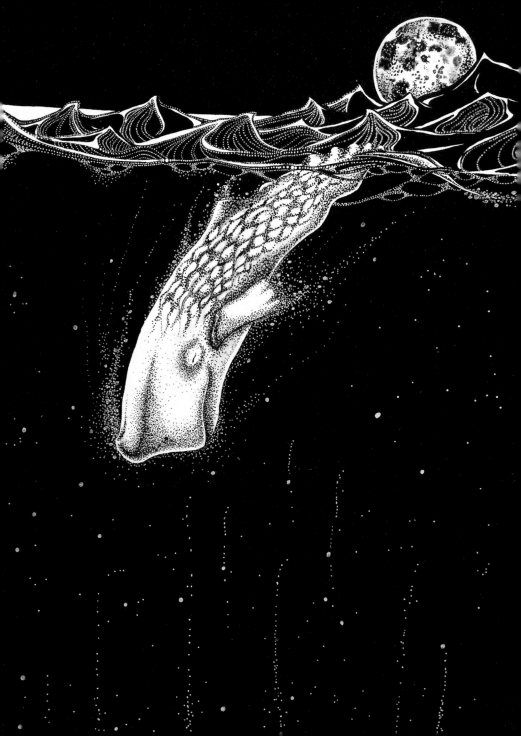

September 1

A PASSENGER SEES a small portion of the ocean from the porthole of a ship. When he goes up to the open deck, he has a greater perspective of the sea. Our perspectives are our windows into the world. The way we choose to see things can create a narrow or broad outlook. What we focus on expands. Our dreams can offer a deeper perspective on our inner world. May your dreams be open and expansive.

September 2

Nothing is worth more than laughter. It is strength
to laugh and to abandon oneself, to be light.
Tragedy is the most ridiculous thing.

—FRIDA KAHLO

HEAVINESS WEIGHS DOWN the soul. Negative emotions bring the soul's vibration down and positive emotions lift them. When there is heaviness in our hearts, a positive thought can alleviate the weight of the intense emotions. Before you drift off to sleep, do a smiling meditation. Close your eyes and smile, taking deep breaths through the nose. Revel in the lightness.

———

September 3

THROUGHOUT THE COUNTRY MEADOW, the trees and grass grow patiently and quietly. As they expand, so does the meadow's size, beauty, and bounty. The larger the meadow, the more animals hide and burrow in the many new spaces they find there. Like the meadow, be patient and steady in your growth. As our lives expand and evolve, so too will grow the spaces within us in which we can dwell and love.

September 4

EVERY PATH LEADS SOMEWHERE; don't get stuck wondering where you are on a map. If something is not going the way you desire, find a way to use this setback as a stepping-stone. Failures lead to successes when we learn from what went wrong. Each mistake can be a step closer to success. People have created many great things because of the lessons learned from failure. Great things are on their way. Create momentum by recognizing the lesson and moving on.

September 5

WHEN THE DAY IS COMPLETE, we turn off the lights as we prepare for bed. The space becomes dark and our senses adjust. When darkness takes over, we cannot rely on our sight. We must use our other senses a bit more to compensate. At times we feel off and find ourselves overcompensating as a reaction. But if we allow the natural adjustment to take place, we can find our balance more quickly.

September 6

TO BE FEARLESS, we need to starve fear. When we feed our fears, they accumulate strength through the attention we give them. Tonight, allow any fears that have accumulated to drift away as you focus your attention elsewhere. Set the stage for beautiful dreams to occur and give your dreams the attention you withdraw from your fears. This new attention will attract the things you dream about. Fearlessness will grow as you recognize the power of manifestation.

September 7

DEEP IN THE SEA, a school of fish gathers and swims with fluid ease. As the fish ride the currents, they find a natural and communal rhythm. In a group they find security traversing the ocean. Our community can be a place of safety and camaraderie. Think about your community this evening and offer gratitude for every member. Notice where the movements of your group are fluid and where you may need to make adjustments. Visualize fluid movements as if you are all riding an ocean current.

September 8

A RUBBER BAND IS STRETCHED and then bounces
back to its former shape. At times we feel stretched
and find it difficult to return to our original state. But our
brains are elastic and have the ability to bend and shape,
depending on what we focus on. If negative thoughts
permeate your mind, you are creating a negative pattern
in your brain. By focusing on positive thoughts, over
time the brain's elasticity will develop positivity where
negativity once resided.

September 9

THROUGH THE CRACKS, light creeps into places that
were once dark. A crack may seem like a defect, but
also a place where beauty is revealed. In the Japanese
tradition of Kintsugi, broken pottery is repaired using
gold. A precious metal replaces the break, creating depth
and beauty. A place that was once broken can develop a
newfound strength and beauty. Embrace your cracks and
look for the loveliness and depth they provide.

September 10

DURING THE STRONGEST WINDS, the branches of a tree sway, giving in to the wind's influence. Down on the ground, the trunk stands firm with its roots reaching into the earth, allowing the branches the freedom to sway. Like a tree, we can find stillness through the changes in life. It is important to stay grounded and find our inner stillness to help get through such times. Find your center and allow stillness to calm and ground you.

September 11

I seem to be waiting for something to happen—
I've tried not to think because there are so many
things that make me feel so exquisitely raw inside.

—GEORGIA O'KEEFFE

ANTICIPATION CAN BE EXCITING as well as anxiety-ridden. When there are many unknown factors, focusing on the wait can deprive you of joy in the present. Whatever is going to happen is already on its way. Infuse the present with positive thoughts and energy so that when the outcome manifests, you will be ready with a positive outlook and a joyful heart.

———

September 12

SHALLOW WATER SITS CALMLY in the tide pool where the starfish rests. The starfish clings to a rock to find stability and balance through the rising tides of the sea. As the tide rises, the water becomes increasingly turbulent and the starfish's grip on the rock keeps the creature in place. When we go through turbulent times, it is important to have a network we can rely on. Offer appreciation for the rocks in your life.

September 13

SEPTEMBER'S HARVEST MOON: Bright in the sky, the moon shines down, providing the light for the harvest. Hard work and patience are rewarded as farmers reap what they sowed in the spring. It is time to reflect on how your seeds have developed. Harvest is the culmination of growth and pruning. Appreciate the work that this harvest provided. Be grateful for your patience and perseverance. Breathe in this contentment and allow your dreams to revel in this harvest.

September 14

AS THE SEASON TURNS from summer to fall, the leaves change colors on trees, adding brightness to a cooler environment. Before they fall, golden leaves—the final burst of sunny color—are a reminder of the summer's vibrancy. When the final leaf falls, the tree becomes dormant in preparation for the winter. This is the perfect time to reflect on your vibrancy. Even during transitions, we emit light. Notice if there are any places where the light has dimmed and infuse vibrancy in that place.

September 15

THE PEOPLE WE SURROUND ourselves with influence the energy we invite into our lives. Take a moment to think about the people who have the most influence on your life. Notice the energy that you associate with each one. If you identify excessive negativity, figure out a way to reverse that energy or stop the exchange all together. Focus on the sources that provide positive energy in your life. Be grateful for the people who infuse your life with happiness and joy. Your energy attracts like-minded individuals.

———

September 16

AN UNBRIDLED HORSE RUNS wild across the plains; its mane flows wildly in the wind as its legs pound the earth in determined fervor. Freedom runs rampant through each muscle. Freedom allows the horse to run miles and gain strength from this independence. When nothing holds us back, it is amazing how far we will go. We compete only against ourselves in the space of freedom. Let your dreams run wild with determination.

September 17

I like living. I have sometimes been wildly, despairingly,
acutely miserable, racked with sorrow, but through it all I still
know quite certainly that just to be alive is a grand thing."
—AGATHA CHRISTIE

LIFE IS BEAUTIFUL. Will all of its pain, suffering, and
ambiguity, there is joy, beauty, and grace all around. The
balance of these extremes creates a beautiful story with
you as the hero, overcoming obstacles and growing in
wisdom.

———

September 18

UP ON THE HEADLANDS, a woman looks out to sea,
searching for migrating whales. She waits patiently
to see them spout. The ocean rewards those who are
patient. The woman sits and looks, knowing that in time
they will arrive. Upon the first sighting, her heart flutters;
she feels as if she is seeing a long-lost love. She reveres
these massive creatures and watches in awe. Whatever
you are waiting for is on its way. Watch in awe and
gratitude when it arrives.

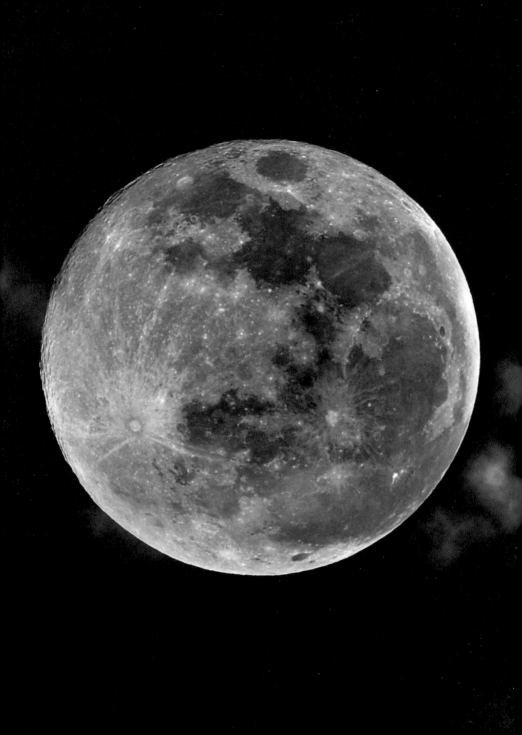

September 19

GRACE IS THE SOFTNESS that brings understanding and love to a difficult situation. It alleviates and creates space for healing. Grace and patience work together to keep balance and love flowing. To offer grace, you need to have a softened heart. When grace arrives, there is no room for resentment or bitterness. It says, "I am here even though I don't need to be." Hold this thought for a moment and offer yourself grace this evening.

September 20

DURING AN EQUINOX, the Earth experiences a balance between daylight and darkness. It is a time to reset the season and move into cooler or warmer weather. Days become shorter or longer. This day of balance can be a personal check-in for inner balance. Do you have equal productivity and rest? Are you eating a balanced diet? Do you provide equal attention to your mind, body, and soul? Take a moment to scan and see where imbalances may be and resolve to regain balance.

September 21

A GREAT REVELATION IS exciting. When you anticipate something, the idea of the unknown and the ability to wait are lovely together. When expectation takes over, patience may wane. Trust and patience work together to keep our minds from trying to control the outcome. If you are waiting for something, revel in the glory of anticipatory joy and rest in patience knowing that in time, all will be revealed.

September 22

I decided, very early on, just to accept life unconditionally;
I never expected it to do anything special for me, yet I
seemed to accomplish far more than I had ever hoped. Most
of the time it just happened to me without my ever seeking it.
—AUDREY HEPBURN

EXPECTATIONS LAY A FOUNDATION for disappointment.
We can accomplish great things when we measure
without expectations. Let go of the outcome and see
the positive in all things, no matter how great or small.
Wonderful things are happening all around us.

September 23

A NEON-BLUE WAVE CRASHES onto the shore in the
middle of the night. Below the surface, an overgrowth
of algae turns the tide into a late-night light show. Under
the moon's soft glow, bioluminescence can mesmerize
us. Perception can turn something simple into something
awe-inspiring. Some things need to be observed in the
dark for us to see their luminous beauty. Look in wonder
often and see loveliness all around. Just below the
surface, anything may reveal its glow.

September 24

We have the capacity to receive messages from
the stars and the songs of the night winds.
—RUTH ST. DENIS

SIT QUIETLY AND EXHALE all the stress from the day. Seek the messages that wait in the stillness. We are connected to the stars and the wind. Locate the place where your intuition resides. Ask a question that is on your mind and wait for the answer. Let go of your timetable. The answer will appear when the timing is right.

———

September 25

A MUSICAL INSTRUMENT becomes a song when a musician puts it to use. The player creates the sounds. A wrong note can create discord in the song. The musician corrects the note and continues to play. When we face discord in our lives, we can be like a musician and continue with the song. We can learn that we do not need to dwell upon missteps, but can recognize them and use them for forward movement.

September 26

WISHES ARE SEEDS for the soul to germinate and manifest. Belief nourishes the wish depending on whether they are positive or negative. If there is a wish that you desire to take place, nurture it with positive thoughts and allow the wish to take the shape it is destined for. Suspend doubt to manifest your desires.

———

September 27

THE MIND CAN SEEM MOST ACTIVE late at night when you most need sleep. To quiet the mind, create a space for stillness. You may feel resistance at first because the brain wants to continue its endless loop— but with persistence, stillness can take over. Begin in a comfortable position and take in a deep breath through your nose and hold it for one count. As you exhale, open your mouth, allowing your breath to be louder than your thoughts. Repeat ten times. Notice the stillness you create with just your breath.

September 28

Life is not a having and a getting, but a being and becoming.
—MYRNA LOY

WE HAVE THE ABILITY to be whatever we want to be. We can become the person we want to become. But too often we allow fear and doubt to take over. We wait for material things to fill voids that only actualized dreams can fulfill. Remember your dreams. Go after what you really want. Tonight, may your dreams be full of success and awe. May you become what you dream of.

———

September 29

AT THE TOP OF A MOUNTAIN, a climber looks down. The rush of accomplishment she feels is accompanied by a sense of personal pride. After months of training, she has reached the mountaintop. Upon descent, the climber knows this is not the last mountain she will climb. We all have summits to ascend in life. Each one holds its own sense of victory. Keep aiming high and scale as many mountains as you can.

September 30

What hurts you blesses you, darkness is your candle.

—RUMI

THE REASON MANY THINGS HAPPEN is unclear until they are behind us. Some challenges are blessings in disguise that keep us from harm, stop a painful pattern, or create an opening to allow what is supposed to happen. Light can come through darkness in the form of wisdom and enlightenment. After a hurt, we are never the same. The scar is the place of healing.

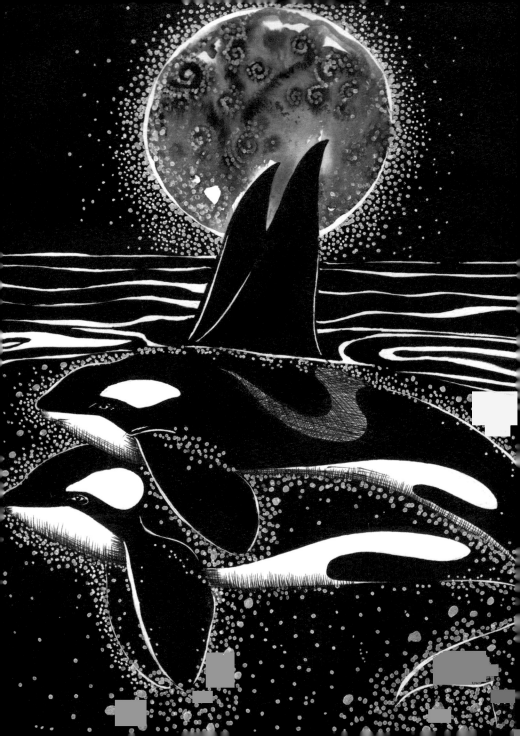

October 1

PAINTBRUSH TO CANVAS. Colors blend. Each stroke creates a new element of depth. There are no mistakes in creativity. An artist builds upon layers as a painting takes shape. At first there may be a cacophony of colors before a masterpiece appears. When we are going through ambiguous times, we may feel directionless and the unknown can cause trepidation. Remember that through the layers, you are making a thing of beauty.

October 2

THE HEARTBEAT IS THE NATURAL rhythm that our souls dance to. We begin life by lying close to our mother's heartbeat and feeling our own meld with hers. We experience our first symphony in the womb and we carry that beat deep inside throughout our lives. To access our primal rhythm, we need to find stillness to connect with our heartbeat. Place your hand over your heart and sync your breath to create a symphony in stillness.

———

October 3

WE ALWAYS HAVE A CHANCE to begin again. Let go of whatever happened today, knowing that tomorrow is new and full of opportunity. Allow yourself to become still and to breathe in this moment. Notice any tension you may be holding on to and breathe soothing breaths into that space. Let the breath melt the tension from your body and feel yourself becoming lighter in the stillness.

October 4

LOOKING UP INTO the infinite vastness of the stars brings attention to the size of the planet where we live. Earth is a small dot in an enormous universe. Galaxies exist light years beyond our perception and understanding. Thinking about this scale reminds us that many of our worries will soon pass. Stars still shine, the Earth still revolves around the sun, and everything is going to be OK. Whatever the trouble, let it go and rest, knowing that life continues beyond our worries.

———

October 5

WATER FLOWS, CREATING constant movement and renewal. As the ocean moves to the shore, earth washes away as it pulls back. When water flows through rocks, it moves part of the rock with it, creating erosion and a new shape. Being in the flow means that we may not end up where we started, but there is a promise of movement and renewal. Imagine yourself as a large wave coming to shore. Now see it washing away the day's troubles and leaving space for the newness of tomorrow.

October 6

Believe there is a great power silently working all things
for good, behave yourself and never mind the rest.

—BEATRIX POTTER

EVERYTHING EVENTUALLY WORKS OUT. The
universe has a grand design, and in that truth we can let
go of the need to control. The only things we can control
are our actions and reactions. Don't worry about others—
they too can control only themselves. Allow the universe
to work things out and take care of your part.

October 7

WHEN FARMERS HARVEST their crops, they celebrate
another year of hard work coming to fruition. Crops vary
in size each year, but growth occurs, and the harvest is
evidence of the farmers' labor. A mind-set of abundance
allows us to plant a seed and imagine it growing,
blossoming, and bearing fruit. When you plant seeds,
approach them with abundance and trust that their needs
are being provided for.

October 8

A SWAN GLIDES ACROSS the water gracefully with its beautiful white feathers and long, slender neck. It is a symbol of grace. Under the surface, its feet paddle to maintain momentum to keep the swan afloat. Grace takes work. It can be difficult to offer forgiveness, love, and acceptance where it may not seem deserved. When grace is needed, think about the swan paddling its feet and accept the work that needs to happen.

———

October 9

SILENCE IS HEALING and can be more powerful than noise. In outer space, there is a void where stars, planets, and moons revolve around the sun. The solar system demonstrates the ability to orchestrate without sound. The most powerful forces in nature coordinate to make this silent symphony take place. If the solar system can operate in silence, we can take a lesson and harness the power of silence. Create a space of sacred silence and just be.

October 10

A SNAKE SHEDS ITS SKIN as it grows, making room for the transformation taking place. Each new skin is a sign of renewal. As we undergo transformations in our mind, body, and soul, we generate a newness and let go of things that no longer serve us. Each shedding clears space for a rebirth and reconciliation. Transformations can be difficult, but the more we surrender to them, the easier they become. Let go of all that holds you back and ease into the renewal that awaits.

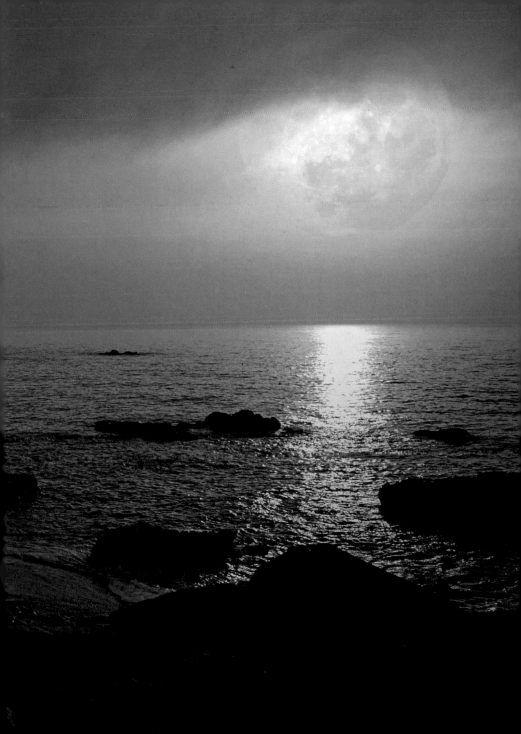

October 11

TIME SLIPS BY WITHOUT NOTICE when we spend our days in a rush. Taking moments to practice mindful awareness creates a sense of pause and calm. Breathe into beautiful moments to take in the sights, sounds, smells, tastes, and feelings they bring. Make mental notes of where you experience awe. Pause in awe. These moments are gratitude generators. Contemplate the beautiful moments of the day and appreciate the awe they provided. Then, breathe in the current moment and recognize its beauty.

October 12

OCTOBER'S HUNTER'S MOON: The hunters walk through the fields the morning after the harvest, noticing hills and gullies that were formerly obscured by waves of crops. Just like the newly harvested fields, our lives can reveal what was once hidden when they are cleared. Is there anything left that you need to harvest or let go of? Now is the time to complete the process of reaping what you sowed in the spring. Breathe in this openness; breathe out any residue that may be left. In this open space, new ideas can be revealed.

October 13

When you get into a tight place and everything goes
against you till it seems as though you could not hang
on a minute longer, *never give up then*, for that is just
the place and time that the tide'll turn.

—HARRIET BEECHER STOWE

TIDES RISE AND FALL and never stay the same. They
leave the shore renewed every time they leave. Don't
give up; renewal and growth are happening, producing a
new level of comfort.

October 14

BECOMING FAMILIAR WITH the night sky and the
currents of the ocean, tribes in the South Pacific drew on
their connection with nature to accomplish the amazing
feat of crossing the sea in a small boat. Constellations led
the way, aiding the explorers on their ocean adventures.
They embraced the unknown, and beautiful islands waited
on the other side. Embrace ambiguity and search for the
beauty that waits on the other side of the unknown.

October 15

AS THE SUN DIPS into the ocean, a surfer looks out to the sea, searching for the perfect wave. The sky turns from pink to lavender and the waves dance amid the changing colors. The ocean is ready to dance with the surfer and carry him or her to and fro. It relaxes, allowing the surfer to glide, then tenses up to lift its wave and deliver the ride the surfer came for. Be like the surfer and be ready to receive.

———

October 16

KINDNESS CREATES CONNECTION and healing. Our words and actions are products of our hearts and soul. What we think and feel manifests outwardly. If you experienced a moment of kindness today, breathe in the fullness of that joy. Remember how it felt to give or receive that kindness. Deposit the feeling into your memory bank so that you can recall it later. Kind thoughts produce kindness. The more we contemplate good things, the more we will exude goodness.

October 17

IN AN ENDING, THERE IS always a beginning. Finishing something creates an opening for something else to take its place. Even in death, the cycle continues as particles return to the Earth to help provide for a new beginning. Everything is connected in a cyclical manner. Honor where you are in this cycle. Give thanks for the cycle of the day and how the sun gave light to the moon as the Earth cycled past it.

———

October 18

DURING A STORM, a snail emerges, moving slowly to avoid drowning. It is not worried about the rain or its pace; it just continues to move forward. Even at the risk of exposure to predators, snails move without fear. When life feels stormy, keep moving forward. One small step each day can create the momentum you need while the storm passes. Don't allow fear to paralyze movement. Keep going, because storms always pass.

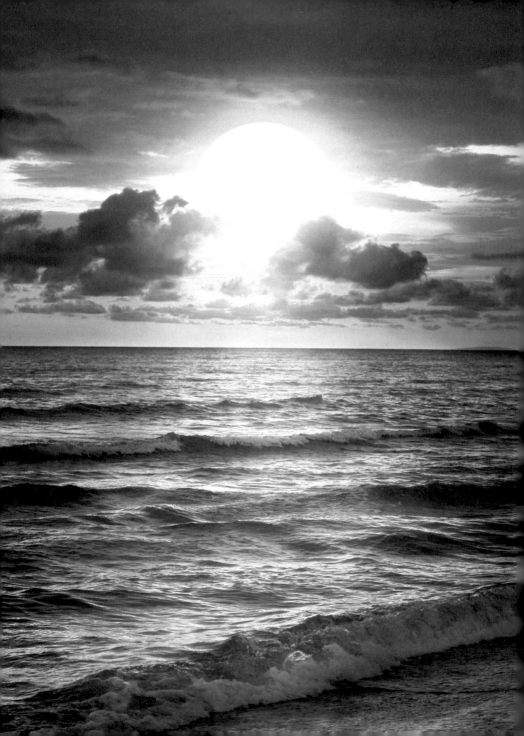

October 19

A STATE OF ABUNDANCE does not mean material
wealth. We have abundance when our physical,
emotional, and spiritual needs are met. Practicing
gratitude invites us to reflect on the ways those needs
have been met. If we operate from a state of abundance,
we notice that just having what we need is a form
of abundance. If thoughts creep in about what you
lack, reframe them into thoughts of sufficiency and, if
possible, abundance. Giving thanks for every little thing
is the key to abundant living.

October 20

INTERRUPTIONS AND unscheduled changes can cause imbalance. Responding to change with a reaction disrupts balance. It is inevitable that plans are interrupted and schedules change. Choosing to be calm during the transition will alleviate stress and encourage equilibrium. Schedules are only guidelines and interruptions need not hold power. Finding your breath in these moments will help ease tension. Breathe in balance; breathe out reactions.

———

October 21

My life didn't please me so I created my life.
—COCO CHANEL

WE HAVE THE POWER to create our reality. If you need to make a change, begin by taking small steps to help create the life you desire. All great things begin with the first step. As you drift off to sleep, create a vision of the change you would like to create. See yourself as if the change has already happened. This is the first step in moving toward your desire.

October 22

THERE ARE INLETS in the coastline that create safe harbors where the wind is not as harsh and the water is calmer. Harbors allow for a break from being out to sea and battling the harsher conditions. Taking breaks is necessary in order to operate at the fullest potential. Find the time to create a safe harbor during hectic times. Allow bedtime to create the calm break from everyday life. Leave life and all its troubles at the door and melt into peaceful sleep.

October 23

A LOTUS RADIATED BEAUTY and noticed how people stopped to admire it. The lotus worried that the admirers would be alarmed if they knew that every night, it descended into the mud only to return the next day. Perfectionism can create discontentment and judgment. What others don't see does not affect them. Self-judgment removes joy from situations where love and acceptance await. Accept what is and offer love and gratitude to those places where acceptance is needed. Without the mud, the lotus would not be as radiant.

October 24

DURING A DROUGHT, scarcity is prevalent. The lack of water creates a mind-set of shortage. Reserving water becomes an important focus, to ensure that the supply lasts. But the rain always appears and the water supply becomes replenished. We experience droughts in the soul when we find ourselves in a mind-set of deficiency and scarcity. To counteract this, focus on what is being supplied right now and remember that the rain always returns

———

October 25

FEARS CAN TAKE OVER when what-if takes root in the soul. It is easy to run through various scenarios that could happen. But those things may never occur, and then the time spent worrying takes away from time that could have been spent at peace. Spend some time listing all your what-ifs and think about how those thoughts and energy can be redirected towards things that are happening right now. Instead of wondering about tomorrow, focus on today.

October 26

A DOLPHIN POD SWIMS parallel to shore, playfully zipping past each other as a large wave begins to accumulate. The closer the wave gets to the shore, the higher the swell becomes. The dolphins adjust their swimming to ride the wave and then continue on their way. Life will send large waves that will throw us off course momentarily. When the wave passes, we can continue on the path or forge a new one. Honor the perspective that arrived during the momentary detour.

———

October 27

EVERYONE HAS THEIR OWN unique struggles. When the pain passes, we are provided with the opportunity to help another person who will face a similar hardship someday. Our struggles can be seen as a gift and a tool to encourage and inspire others. Honor the struggle by offering gratitude for the lesson and perspective it provided. Your soul guided you through and that energy will help someone find your inspiration just when they need it. The healed can become the healer.

October 28

Look at how a single candle can both defy
and define the darkness.

—ANNE FRANK

WITHOUT LIGHT, DARKNESS would not be noticed. Without darkness, light would not be seen. When we shine from within, we can illuminate our souls as well as recognize where our darkness has seeped back in. This illumination is a gift. Embrace the darkness and see how you are changing the lighter you shine. You can choose to shine, even when darkness is present.

———

October 29

EXPECTATIONS SET US up for disappointments. When we expect something from a person, place, or experience, we often find ourselves dissatisfied and frustrated. We cannot rely on something outside of ourselves to bring fulfillment; that comes from within. Understanding that each encounter offers the opportunity for growth can bring us back to the present moment. Abandon expectations and practice being present.

October 30

THE PILGRIM MOVES FORWARD each day in search
for spiritual awakening and inspiration. Roads seem to go
on forever and during the journey, doubt can take over.
On the way, many different people and emotions are
met. Some stay with the pilgrim and others only create
a barrier from the path. At the end of the journey, the
pilgrim realizes that everything happened for a reason
and each instance made him stronger and more resilient.

———

October 31

IMAGINE YOU ARE SITTING on a cliff overlooking the
ocean. Feel the sun shining down on you. As you watch
the waves rise and fall, you become very still and notice
this sense of peace is with you always as you breathe
into the present moment. You close your eyes and allow
the ocean's song to create a rhythmic calm within. Your
breath becomes one with the waves. As thoughts enter,
they leave just as a wave breaks. Breathe in peace;
breathe out everything else.

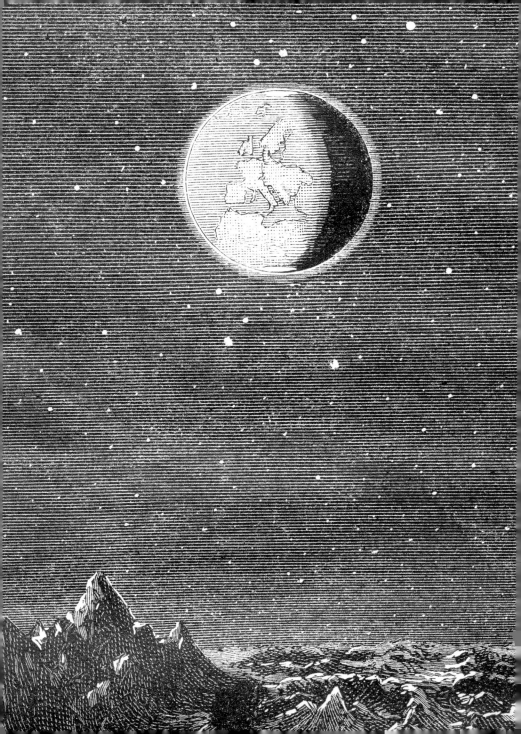

November 1

TO LOVE SOMEONE MEANS that you do not expect anything in return. Love is one of the most basic human needs. We desire the love of others and when our hearts are open we wish to give love. Keeping the heart open is essential to nurture and extend love. What's most important is to give this gift to ourselves. When we can love ourselves, we can love others. As you fall asleep, reflect on all of the things you love about yourself.

November 2

WITHIN THE TEARS of frustration is the release of letting go. Frustration occurs when we realize that the control we desire is not attainable. Releasing our attachment to the outcome and offering an open mind and heart to the situation creates grace and patience. Sometimes knowing is not the goal. Release your grasp on the road map you are determined to use; a better plan is in the works. Trust the process.

———

November 3

TO ACT OUT OF LOVE is to act from a vulnerable place where the heart is open and ready to give. Keeping the heart open and giving love is a great feat. When we do small things from this place of openness and love, it changes the giver and the receiver. Imagine if we each did one small thing every day with love from our open hearts.

November 4

STILLNESS INVITES things to come mentally and physically. Frantically going about life can leave little room for invitations and explorations. Finding a place of inner calm brings moments of clarity and attracts opportunities. At the end of each day, take the time to pause and reflect. Let go of any troubles that occurred during the day. Open the mind to the lesson that arose and be grateful for what transpired.

November 5

A HARDENED HEART can soften again with enough care and love. Trials and fire soften some of the hardest and densest materials and souls. Forgive and heal whatever caused the hardness. Allow grace to enter the space that has atrophied. Let grace permeate the space and slowly reveal and soften the core where love and understanding reside. In this space, forgiveness and love can return and heal. Embrace the release. Soften into restoration.

November 6

OUR FIRST RELATIONSHIPS are with our mothers in the womb. We bond before we are even born, connecting on a physical level. By being born, we are transformed from dependent to independent, able to breathe on our own. As we grow up, we become completely independent. This evening, think of the earth as your mother, and thank her for nurturing you. Offer gratitude for the life, lessons, and kindness she has offered.

November 7

Why turn your eyes to your shadow, when, by looking upward, you see your rainbow in the same direction?
—MARIA MITCHELL

WHEN WE LOOK DOWN after a rainstorm, we become aware of puddles. Stepping over a puddle can keep you from getting wet. But if we look up, we might witness rainbows and clouds. If we are always looking for what may cause discomfort, we will miss the things that can bring us awe. By avoiding discomfort, we may deprive ourselves of beauty and wonder.

November 8

PELICANS GLIDE OVER THE OCEAN in formation looking for food. Their flight patterns are effortless and graceful. They change direction with the wind, letting the currents guide the way. They follow their prey from above, waiting for the perfect time to dive down. By keeping a distance from their goal, they can find the best opportunity to act. Whenever we face a goal, we can be like a pelican and rise above it to find the best timing for action. By stepping back, we gain perspective.

November 9

WHEN THE EVENING AIR becomes crisp in autumn, the harvest is almost complete. Fruit and grain are gathered after a bountiful growing season. The work of pruning in the spring and tending in the summer determines the quality of the crop. At times, there are plants that will not produce, so they are no longer tended to. If there is something that does not promise growth, focus elsewhere. Reaping what we sow also applies to the attention that we give. Place your attention on areas of growth.

November 10

THINGS COME TO AN END for a reason. Death is not only an ending but also a beginning. When a flower dies, it falls to the ground and creates room for another bloom to occur. If something in your life is ending, let go and make room for what wants to come. Open your heart and mind to whatever is next. The pain of the ending will pass and the beauty and joy of a new beginning will replace it.

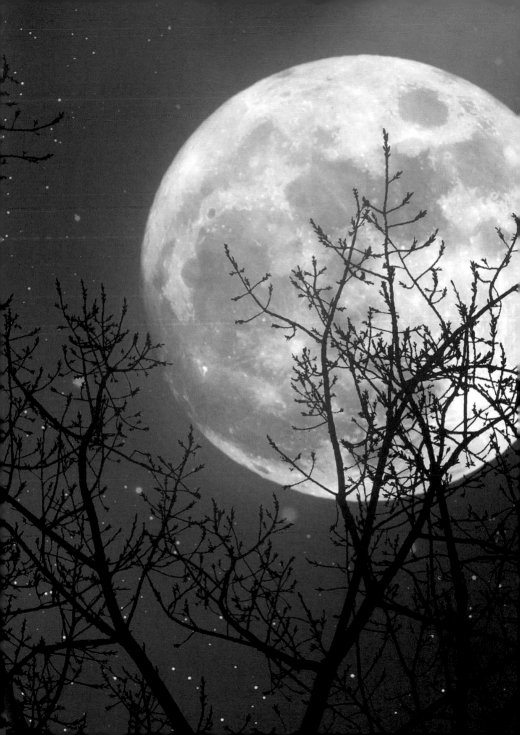

November 11

A SAPLING SPLIT IN THE CENTER, creating two trees from a single growth. Some things grow together for a time and then branch off to grow apart. What once thrived together now thrives apart. At times what we intend to grow does not produce what we had imagined. Our efforts can make something else occur and we can either embrace it or reject it. If the tree is split and thriving on its own, let it be. Don't force things to happen.

November 12

EVERY SNOWFLAKE IS DIFFERENT and significant. Each one eventually delivers water to streams and lakes. We can behold wonder and beauty in such a small thing. Each human is different and significant as well. Each person has a purpose and a soul. Looking for the beauty in every person we meet fosters acceptance and tolerance. Offer the love and appreciation you desire to others. Genuinely embrace differences. Where there is acceptance there is peace and understanding.

November 13

NOVEMBER'S BEAVER MOON: To prepare for the bareness of winter, a beaver gathers and builds a safe, warm place. Many animals collect their reserves for hibernation. This is the time for preparation and planning. What are you preparing and planning for? If you would like to get something done, create a plan. Allow your dreams to take place in this sacred space. Don't force anything. Breathe in this openness and breathe out worry. Everything will fall into place.

November 14

THE VASTNESS OF SPACE is a place where anything is possible and galaxies exist. Comets fly, planets orbit the sun, and stars are born. Creating spaciousness in our minds and in our physical environments makes room for stillness and peace. We can realize and actualize greatness in the space of stillness. A quiet mind is like a clean, blank page. Contemplate possibility. Allow dreams to take place. There are no boundaries where creation awaits.

November 15

WHEN FEAR SPEAKS, it repeats untruths you have told yourself over the years. We listen to fear in our most vulnerable states, especially when something is at risk. Don't let fear talk you out of something amazing and beautiful. Stop it in its tracks and tell the truth. Notice what is really going on and let fear dissipate as truth permeates your mind. Recognize your vulnerability and embrace your tenderness. Allow truth to fuel your courage.

———

November 16

THE ART OF DOING NOTHING cultivates great understanding. When our minds are full of thoughts and our days are busy, understanding does not have room to expand. Find some time each day to stop for a few minutes to breathe and clear space. When you first wake up, take five breaths to ground yourself. In the middle of the day, take five breaths to regroup. At the end of the day, take five breaths to calm down. Extend the stillness as time goes on.

November 17

A TETHERED HORSE DREAMED of running wild as his soul yearned to be free. Every day he waited for his moment to run free, feeling the wind in his mane, liberated. Days passed and his patience waxed and waned like the pull of the moon. He knew his day was coming. He knew his legs would feel the freedom of running. The day he broke free was the day his soul aligned. Don't ignore your soul's tugs; alignment is waiting.

———

November 18

*All these things must come to the soul from
its roots, from where it is planted.*
—SAINT TERESA OF ÁVILA

ROOTS HOLD PLANTS and trees in place. They dig deep into the earth, creating support for what is above ground. An entirely unseen network thrives beneath the tallest trees and the most beautiful flowers. Without roots, the tree would fall and the flower would shrivel. Our thoughts root us. Our actions and energy nurture what we have planted.

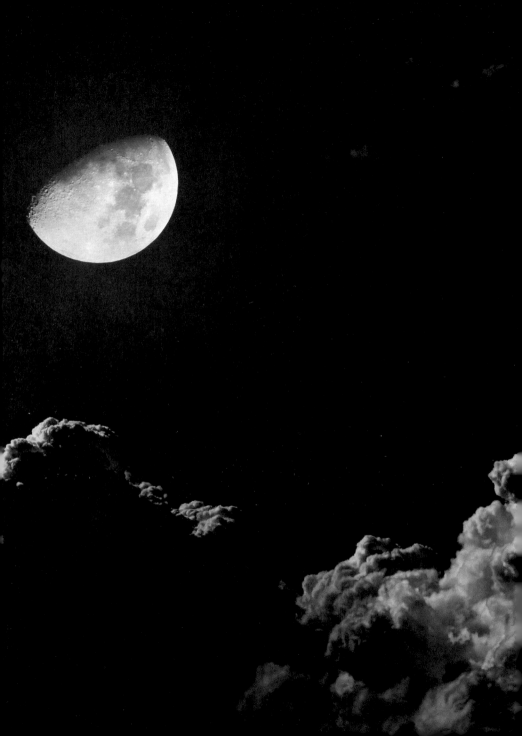

November 19

WATERFALLS ARE MAJESTIC to behold. A rush of
water tumbles down the side of a mountain into a stream
or river below. Approaching the waterfall, you can feel its
energy and power. Behind it there is a peace. Through
the water, you can see the direction; the perspective is
clearer. The same could be said about tears. When they
rush through, there is power and intensity in the feeling.
But on the other side of our tears, after the release, we
can see more clearly.

November 20

WOMEN CARRY BASKETS on their heads on their way to a temple. Inside they make an offering to their gods. Their practice is reverent. They provide offerings that represent faith and respect, no matter what they have to give. Every day we have the opportunity to provide an offering to ourselves, the universe, and others. We can offer positivity, kindness, love, and peace. It is up to you to decide what you will offer each day. Search your heart to learn what it wants to extend to yourself and others.

———

November 21

FEELING WORTHY COMES from deep within. When we feel worthy, we love better, give wholeheartedly, and are more vibrant. Start by noticing how we value ourselves. To accept great things, we need to believe that we deserve them. Take a moment to acknowledge your greatness and your potential. See your worth and embrace it. Offer it to yourself and then extend it to others.

November 22

DURING TIMES OF UNCERTAINTY, it is important to stay grounded in things that are certain. We will always want to explore the unknown. Still, some absolute truths can keep us grounded during vague times. Think about the things that have stayed true and the beliefs you hold on to. Find comfort in their unwavering power. The unknown will soon become known, generating a new level of understanding and insight.

———

November 23

BEING IN THE PRESENCE of wonder creates goose bumps and chills up and down the spine. Awe is a place of reverence and inspiration. Countless places and things can amaze and move us at a soul level: the top of a mountain, the end of a race, the birth of a child, the delivery of good news. Life is beautiful this way, delicately tucking wonder away and revealing it just in time for our souls to bow in gratitude.

November 24

A BUOY REMAINS STEADFAST near the harbor, regardless of the conditions of the waves. It bobs back and forth, always returning to its upright position. Birds land on it and waves crash into it—and yet it protects the harbor by creating a boundary. When life crashes down and people come and go, we can remain steadfast by creating boundaries to protect our hearts. Even when the harshest conditions arise, we can be like a buoy and lean back in order to rebound to a stance of strength.

November 25

What is the good of your stars and trees, your sunrise and the wind, if they do not enter into our daily lives?
—E. M. FORSTER

WE HAVE THE OPPORTUNITY to see beauty in everything. We live on a beautiful planet with mountains, trees, sunrises, and shooting stars. Even in the city, we can see beauty in every passing face. Focus on what is beautiful and soon you will notice that it resides in unexpected places.

November 26

IMAGINE THAT YOU ARE near the beach and the water
is calm and warm. Walk out into the ocean and notice
how clear the water is. There is soft white sand at your
feet and warm turquoise water all around. Lie back into
the sea and face the sun. Allow the saltwater to hold your
body. Float effortlessly. Feel the gentle sway of the water
creating immense calm within. As you close your eyes in
bed tonight, recall this image and fall into a deep sleep.

November 27

A SPIDER WEAVES an intricate web under the moonlight
with great care. The creature displays its creativity
while making a place to provide nourishment. Its artistic
instinct is critical to its survival and it weaves the delicate
web with strength and purpose. The spider does not
seek praise; it creates because it must. When expressed,
creativity nourishes the mind, body, and soul. We gain
inner strength by vulnerably displaying the creative spark
that lives inside us.

November 28

AFTER THE FULL MOON, the light wanes, creating a crescent that slowly shades the moon in darkness. During the waning moon cycle, allow closure to take place. Each moon cycle is a time for growth. Soon the time to plant will return. But for now, close the doors that need to shut. Another beginning is just around the corner. Prepare the space for whatever is next.

———

November 29

PAIN CAN FEEL AS DEEP as the ocean. Sorrow can take us far into the depths, where nothing can reach us. But there is life in the depths. The ocean is full of vibrant life; new creatures are still being discovered. In the depths, life is still happening and something new is being discovered. Contemplate in this quiet place. Find the sliver of hope, like a moonbeam that permeates the sea, and use it as a beacon as you make your way back to the surface.

November 30

A TRANQUIL SEA reflects like glass. In the stillness of
the sea, the sky can see its reflection on the water and
admire its own vast beauty. There is nothing disrupting
the placid scene as serenity takes over. When the sky is
turbulent with storms, the sea reflects the energy with
the tossing and turning of its waves. Similarly, we reflect
the energy we emit. Give off the energy you want to
receive and abide in.

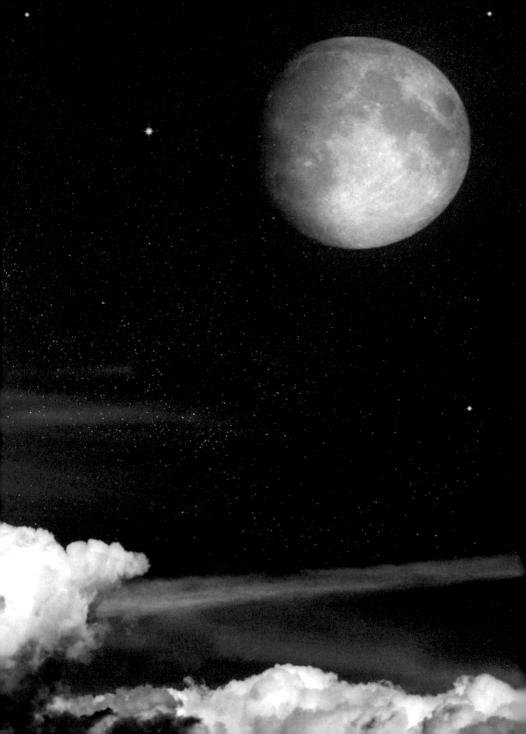

December 1

A MOTH'S ACTIVITIES ARE CONDUCTED at night.
The moth navigates using the moon's light. Naturally
attracted to light, moths are drawn to lamps and fires
as well. Their attraction to light makes them seem
mysterious when they appear from the dark. They bring
with them vital nectar to pollinate plants and flowers to
help keep nature's balance. The light guides them and
helps their journey. Even when the moon is new, a moth
always finds light to help it on its way.

December 2

EACH OF US HAS an inner compass that guides us and pulls us. If we choose to listen to this guide, we can experience life in a way that is more in tune with nature on an organic level. Our intuition tugs at our soul like the moon with the tides, gently pulling the water closer to and farther from the shore. Locate your truth center by recognizing the unmistakable pull of just knowing in your body when something is right or wrong.

———

December 3

NIGHT HAS FALLEN, the stars appear, and the moon creates a silver glow. It is time to rest and renew the mind. Find inner calm by shutting down all devices and giving the body and mind the time to slow down and ease into a restful state. Release everything that happened today. Let go of tomorrow's plans. Set the stage for dreams to occur. Anything is possible in this calm state.

December 4

THE MOON IS ALWAYS PRESENT, even when it is not reflecting the light of the sun. Its presence has steadily continued, seeing all that transpires in the dark. Even on the darkest nights, we can trust that the moon's light will return in an ever-growing crescent. When darkness seems to prevail, trust that light will return. Illuminate the moment with gratitude. Let trust calm your mind as you rest.

———

December 5

THE MOON IS CYCLICAL and reveals in the darkness when she is new. Her light emerges as her crescent waxes, revealing her beauty incrementally. Her regeneration symbolizes hope and new beginnings. When she is full, she shines in all her glory, reflecting the radiance of the sun. She births ideas and encourages creativity. Then her light wanes as she surrenders to the outcome of her intentions. Her light fades, completing a cycle of manifestation.

December 6

I RELEASE ALL THE STRESS from the day and allow calm to permeate my soul. As I breathe in, I bring peace and tranquility to the places that feel tense. As I exhale, I let go of the tension, stress, and frustration. I welcome quiet and surrender any noises in my mind. Rest is the state I am about to enter. Dreams and restoration will come to me in sleep. I breathe in restoration and breathe out the rest of the day.

———

December 7

A FIRE CRACKLES, soup is simmering, and home brings a state of comfort and contentment. Outside the air is cold and the trees are bare. Winter is setting in. Comfort comes in many forms. During the winter, it can be a warm fire, just as a cool breeze can create comfort in the heat of summer. A sense of peace generates comfort and invites contentment. Drift off to sleep with a feeling of peace.

December 8

"Be patient toward all that is unsolved in your heart
and try to love the questions themselves."
– RANIER MARIA RILKE

RELIEF COMES AFTER A TRIAL. The anticipation can be joyful, and our questions do not need to be met with anxiety. Think about a time when you wondered about an outcome. In the moments of waiting, you were growing and preparing for what was next. Take this time to grow in preparation and allow the wait to be filled with joyful excitement. Soon your heart will know the answer.

———

December 9

AFTER MONTHS AT SEA, a boat is approached by a seagull. The crew realizes in relief that the shore is near. This realization renews hope. Although the crew knew the shore would soon appear, the storms and tossing of the sea made them lose hope. It sometimes feels as if there is no end to our troubles. Just when we feel that there is no hope left, something happens and the journey makes sense. Keep going; the shore will appear.

December 10

DRIVING THROUGH THE DESERT can seem long and tedious. We look at the horizon, where sand, cacti, and the sky stretch on for what seems like an eternity. Suddenly a roadrunner whizzes by on the road, providing a welcome break in the monotony. The driver gasps in excitement and smiles at the discovery. Roadrunners are a reminder to be lighthearted. The perception of a boring ride is transformed by the anticipation of discovery. Perception creates awareness.

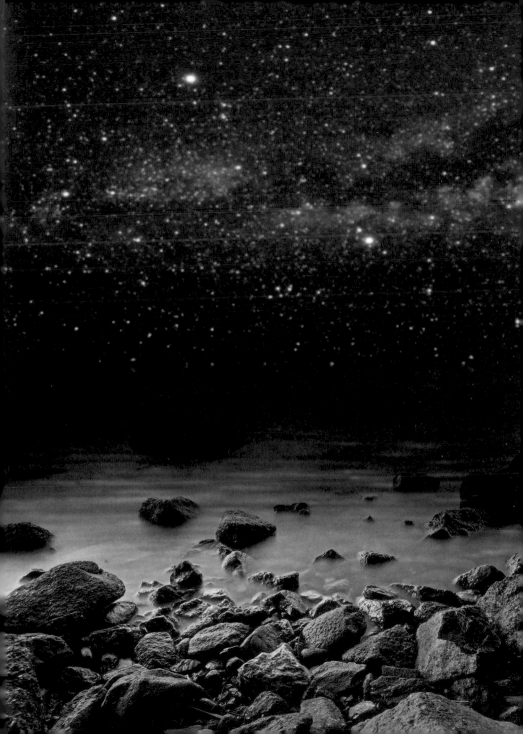

December 11

LOOKING AT A PAINTING close up, you can see
the fine details the painter took to create the scene.
Brushstrokes, blending colors, and fine lines are some of
the small details that make up the big picture. Standing
back, we can view the painter's vision; the perspective
changes and the little things are not as visible. Every
process has fine details we cannot see, but they
contribute to the bigger picture. Perspective depends on
where you stand in the process.

———

December 12

AS THE SUN DIPS BELOW the surface, shadows
are cast, creating silhouettes of the mountains. The
mountains are lit from behind as the sun's final light
emits a fiery orange and pink glow, setting the stage for
the cool light of the moon and stars. There is always light
from above. Even the shadows see the light eventually.
As the Earth makes its way around the sun, all of its
parts become illuminated.

December 13

DECEMBER'S COLD MOON: Deep sleep. Warm bed. Hibernation time. Winter is setting in, the air has become colder, and the days are getting shorter. After the seasons of planting, growth, and harvest, it is time to settle in for rest. Winter provides the time for recovery and reflection. There is nothing left to plan. Let all your troubles slip away as you lie down to sleep. Offer gratitude for a year full of lessons and blessings.

December 14

IN THE DARKNESS OF NIGHT, a nightingale sings its song. He waits for the perfect time to sing—without the noise of other birds—and sings a song for dreamers. Its melody stirs creative potential within the dreamer and releases the mind from the day's troubles. The song is a lullaby that accompanies the shining of the stars. The moon creates a spotlight for the night's song and accompanies it with peace.

December 15

There is something haunting in the light of the moon;
it has all the dispassionateness of a disembodied soul,
and something of its inconceivable mystery.

—JOSEPH CONRAD

THE MOON'S GLOW ILLUMINATES the dark, casts shadows, waxes and wanes. The ever-changing nature of its light moves migrations and tides. It is a reflection of a greater light, yet still holds otherworldly power. You can feel the moon's pull standing underneath its mysterious presence. As it rotates, so does life.

December 16

OXYGEN CREATES A MAGICAL EFFECT on rocks, changing the colors of the minerals within. Reds, yellows, greens, and blues seep through layers of mountainsides, displaying each mineral's hidden beauty. Each layer tells a story of pressure and exposure the rock endured. Through the hardship and change, a rainbow of beauty was formed. Pressure can be the catalyst to a beautiful transformation. Breathe into it and allow change to occur.

December 17

THE BEAUTY OF THE PRESENT MOMENT is that the past is a teacher and the future is a dream. The ability to be right here, right now is a practice. When the lessons or dreams seek attention in the present moment, acknowledge their presence, but let them flow away for they do not have a place right now. Release attachment to outcomes of the past and future and breathe into this moment. Notice something lovely in your surroundings. Pay attention to your breath. Be grateful for the quiet moment you have created for yourself.

December 18

A TREE MAKES ITS WAY through a crevice on a mountainside. Its roots find stability deep within the rocks. Wind blows through the mountaintops, yet the tree remains, growing through the harsh conditions. The roots hold tight and grow stronger with each blast of wind. The trunk twists and turns, creating a stronger anchor, and the green reveals the tree's vitality. Harsh conditions create resilience and strength. Find stability in the roots and continue to reach for the sky.

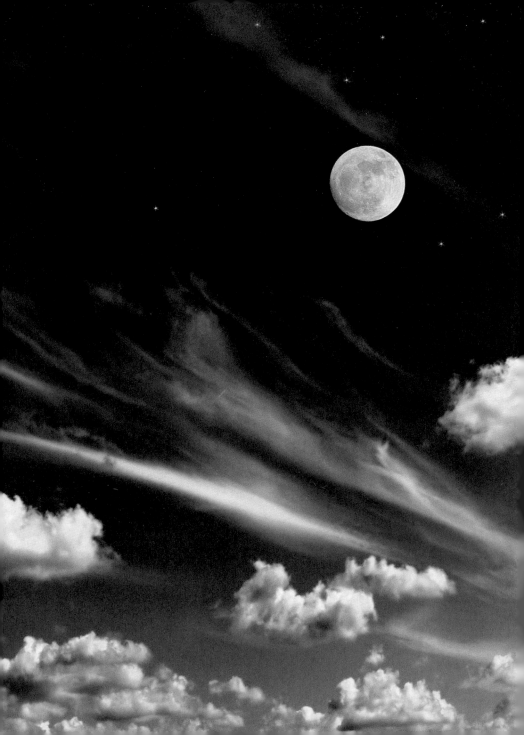

December 19

CORAL IS THE SKELETAL outside of tiny sea creatures; it also creates a home for fish and provides protection for them to hide from predators. The reefs produce a colorful underwater shelf displaying a rainbow of colors. But coral is sharp, and if touched, inflicts pain. The dichotomy of providing protection while inflicting pain highlights its dual nature. Duality exists in all things and we have the power to choose how we perceive them. Perception shapes our reality. Choose to focus on beauty.

December 20

SLUMBER DESCENDS. The body relaxes deeply, releasing all of the tension from the day. There is nothing that needs to be done, no words left to speak. The moon is high in the sky and the stars are dancing in her iridescent light. Lights are dim and the darkness envelops its surroundings like a peaceful hug. Calmness and tranquility manifest through our breath. Dreams unveil themselves from thoughts that are now asleep. Rest takes over.

December 21

DON'T ALLOW OTHERS TO TAKE your power from you. When you find yourself in a situation in which your power is thwarted, stand tall and harness your inner strength. Even when the battle is lost, a remnant of strength still lies deep within. Find your power within and affirm yourself. When you experience a loss or failure, allow it to generate more wisdom to fuel your inner flame. When you can use a loss as fuel, you can shine brighter.

December 22

There are two ways of spreading light; to be
the candle or the mirror that reflects it.

—EDITH WHARTON

THE SUN SHINES BRIGHTLY and its light never
diminishes. The moon is a mirror of the sun at night,
reflecting the sun's brightness during the darkness.
When we shine, our light is reflected in our words,
deeds, and the company we keep. When we have
dimmer days, the light in those around us can help lift us.
We can reflect their brightness when darkness occurs.
There is always light.

December 23

NIGHT IS THE TIME for reflection and rest. The day
is done and regardless of whether you completed
everything, it is time to calm the mind for sleep. Begin
by letting go of the to-do lists and schedule of the day to
come. When tomorrow begins, let your thoughts return
to the day. For now, focus on closing your eyes and
letting go of all thoughts and concerns. Breathe into this
space to make room for dreams.

December 24

SOFT, FLUID, IRIDESCENT, and ever changing, a jellyfish surrenders to the ocean's drifts and currents. As the ocean pushes and pulls, the jellyfish becomes malleable. By letting go, it gets to where it needs to go. It softens against the might of the powerful sea. By softening, difficulties fade away. We can learn a lesson from the jellyfish: Soften, let go, be patient, and you will get where you need to go. Surrender is powerful.

———

December 25

*I must be a mermaid. I have no fear of depths
and a great fear of shallow living.*

—ANAÏS NIN

IN THE DEPTHS, life is abundant and full. Trust, resilience, honesty, compassion, hope, and love reside in the deepest parts of our souls. To find this part of ourselves and others, we must dive deep into conversations, have the encounters that produce growth, and sit in discomfort with each other. There is a level of comfort that only depth can create.

December 26

THE ENDLESS SEARCH for paradise creates a myth that we must discover another place. Paradise is the place where harmony and pleasure exist, where there is no conflict. True paradise can be found within. When the search turns inward, we find treasure because we carry it within. We have a treasure map hidden in our souls and the only way to reach it is through mindfulness and stillness. Search within and find the treasure that has been with you all along.

———

December 27

A WANDERER'S HEART FINDS fulfillment in the journey to the unknown. It is fed by the ever-changing possibilities of discovery, both inward and outward. Nature is full of wandering hearts, as evidenced by the migrations of whales and birds. Home stays with these creatures as they traverse thousands of miles every year. To wander does not mean to be without a home. Home is a place where we find comfort, no matter where the road leads.

December 28

She quietly expected great things to happen to her,
and no doubt that's one of the reasons why they did.

—ZELDA FITZGERALD

OUR THOUGHTS CREATE our reality. If we think
positive thoughts, we attract positive experiences. When
dreams come true, it is because we gave them enough
attention and took action. Notice where your thoughts are
and focus on where you would like to expand.

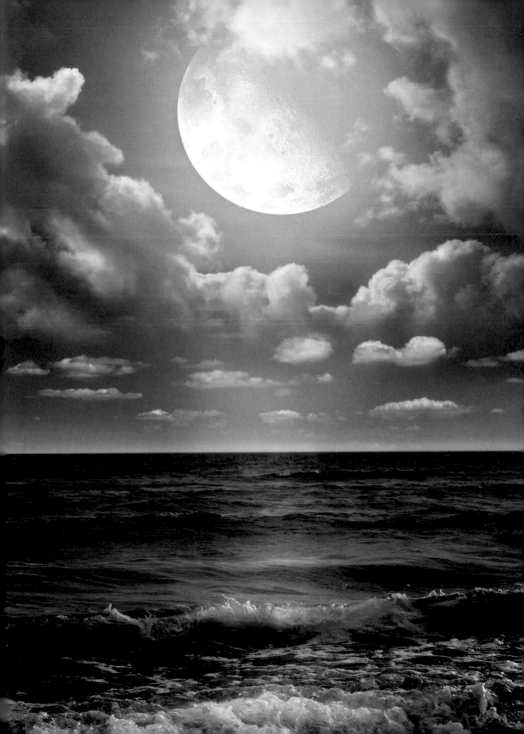

December 29

RIVERS FLOW THROUGH valleys and over places where erosion has created a place to flow. In a river, the continual churning of the water makes rocks smooth. The water's powerful force refines what once had jagged edges. Life's lessons have a tendency to refine us as they repeat until we learn them. Rough edges soften into growth; tenderness occurs where hardness once was.

———

December 30

AT THE BRINK OF FINISHING a goal, an anticipatory excitement often arises. The more clearly the end is in sight, the harder focus may become. It is exciting to know that we are about to achieve something, but as a runner in a race knows, the last stretch is just as important as the first. Whatever you are about to complete, approach the end with integrity. The finished product is a testament to your soul's work.

December 31

LIE DOWN AND BREATHE calming breaths in and out.
Allow the mind to gently become quieter with each
breath. Imagine a calming light emanating from your core
and extending to the edges of your body. Allow this light
to calm any areas of tension and melt away stress. Create
the space for tranquillity and stillness. Let all of the day's
troubles and any residue subside. Sleep is a sacred place
where our subconscious speaks through dreams.

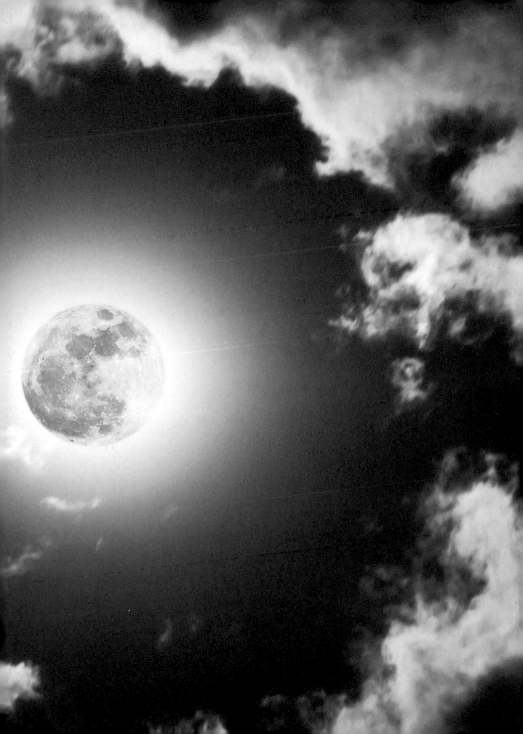

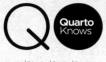

Brimming with creative inspiration, how-to projects, and useful
information to enrich your everyday life, Quarto Knows is a favorite
destination for those pursuing their interests and passions. Visit our
site and dig deeper with our books into your area of interest:
Quarto Creates, Quarto Cooks, Quarto Homes, Quarto Lives,
Quarto Drives, Quarto Explores, Quarto Gifts, or Quarto Kids.

First published in 2017 by Rock Point, an imprint of The Quarto Group,
142 West 36th Street, 4th Floor, New York, NY 10018, USA
T (212) 779-4972 F (212) 779-6058 www.QuartoKnows.com

Rock Point titles are also available at discount for retail, wholesale, promotional, and bulk purchase.
For details, contact the Special Sales Manager by email at specialsales@quarto.com or by mail
at The Quarto Group, Attn: Special Sales Manager, 401 Second Avenue North, Suite 310,
Minneapolis, MN 55401, USA.

10 9 8 7 6 5

ISBN: 978-1-63106-292-6

Art Direction: Merideth Harte
Cover and Interior Design: Yeon Kim

Printed in China

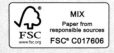

MIX
Paper from
responsible sources
FSC® C017606
FSC
www.fsc.org